Understanding Bipolar Disorder

A Guide to Managing and Living with Mood Swings

Kian M. Hart

Xspurts.com

A New Zealand Designed Product

Other Versions Available

Why limit yourself to just one format?

This book is now available in physical, digital, and audiobook options.

Choose the way you love to read and dive into the story today. You won't regret it!

Digital ISBN: 9781776848126
Physical ISBN: 9781776847037
Audio ISBN:

To obtain a different format of this book at a discounted price, please get in touch with us at:

http://isbn.xspurts.com/

Contents

Have Questions / Comments?

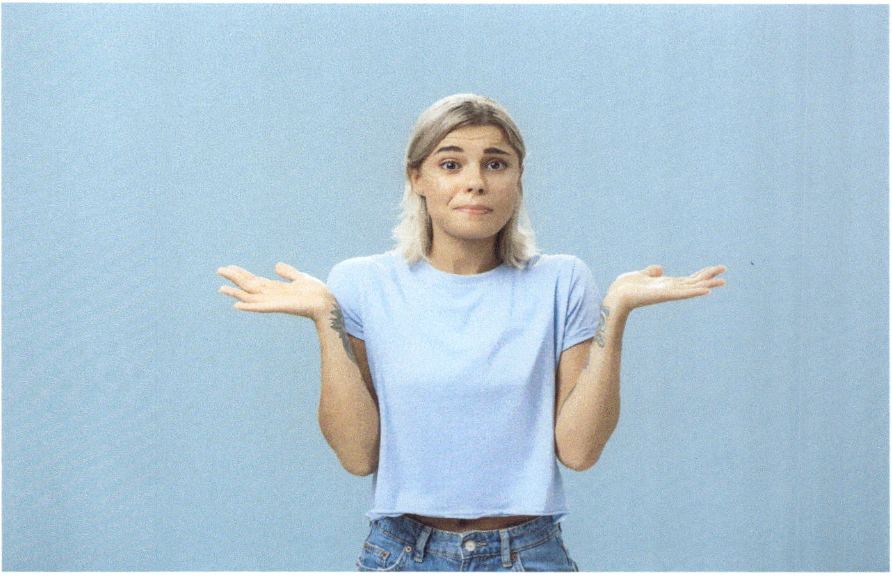

This book was designed to cover as much information as possible, but I know I have probably missed something, or some new amazing discovery has just come out.

If you notice something missing or have a question that I failed to answer, please get in touch and let me know. If I can, I will email you an answer and also update the book so others can also benefit from it.

Thanks For Being Awesome :)

Submit Your Questions / Comments At:

https://questions.xspurts.com

Get Free Stuff

We love writing and have produced a huge number of books.

For being one of our amazing readers, we would love to offer you more books we have created, 100% free.

To claim this limited time special offer, simply go to the site below and enter your name and email address.

You will then receive loads (as we love our readers so much :) of our great books, content and audio direct to your email account, 100% free!

Get Loads of FREE Stuff at:

https://free.xspurts.com

Chapter One

Understanding Bipolar Disorders

Bipolar disorder is a complex mental health condition that affects millions of individuals worldwide. It is characterized by extreme mood swings, ranging from manic highs to depressive lows. These mood episodes can significantly disrupt a person's life, impacting their relationships, work, and overall well, being. Understanding bipolar disorder is crucial for promoting accurate diagnosis, effective treatment, and support for those living with this condition.

One of the key aspects of bipolar disorder is the presence of two distinct mood states: mania and depression. Manic episodes are characterized by an elevated mood, increased energy levels, racing thoughts, and impulsive behavior. Individuals experiencing mania may exhibit grandiose ideas, engage in risky activities, and have a decreased need for sleep. On the other hand, depressive episodes involve persistent feelings of sadness, low energy, loss of interest in previously enjoyed activities, and difficulty concentrating. These mood swings can occur in cycles, with periods of stability in between, or they may manifest as mixed episodes, combining symptoms of both mania and depression.

Bipolar disorder can have a significant impact on a person's life. During manic episodes, individuals may engage in reckless behaviors, such as excessive spending, substance abuse, or risky sexual activities. They may also experience difficulties at work or in relationships due to their erratic behavior and impulsive decision, making. Depressive episodes can lead to feelings of hopelessness, social withdrawal, and even thoughts of self, harm or suicide. It is important to note that bipolar disorder is a chronic condition that requires ongoing management and support.

The exact cause of bipolar disorder is not yet fully understood. However, researchers believe that a combination of genetic, biological, and environmental factors contribute to its development. Studies have shown that individuals with a family history of bipolar disorder are more likely to develop the condition themselves. Imbalances in certain brain chemicals, such as serotonin and dopamine, are also thought to play a role in the development of bipolar disorder. Additionally, stressful life events, substance abuse, and disruptions in circadian rhythms can trigger or exacerbate episodes in susceptible individuals.

Diagnosing bipolar disorder can be challenging due to the variability of symptoms and the overlap with other mental health conditions. A thorough psychiatric evaluation is necessary to rule out other possible causes of mood swings and to determine the presence of distinct manic and depressive episodes. Healthcare professionals rely on the criteria outlined in the Diagnostic and Statistical Manual of Mental Disorders (DSM, 5) to make an accurate diagnosis. It is essential to differentiate bipolar disorder from conditions like major depressive disorder or cyclothymic disorder, as the treatment approaches may differ.

Treatment for bipolar disorder typically involves a combination of medication, psychotherapy, and lifestyle adjustments. Mood stabilizers, such as lithium or anticonvulsant medications, are commonly prescribed to help manage mood swings and prevent relapses. Antidepressants may be used cautiously during depressive episodes, as they can potentially trigger a manic episode. Psychotherapy, such as cognitive, behavioral therapy (CBT) or interpersonal therapy, can be beneficial in helping individuals cope with the challenges of living with bipolar disorder and develop strategies to manage their symptoms. Lifestyle factors, such as maintaining a regular sleep schedule, engaging in regular exercise, and minimizing stress, can also contribute to symptom management.

Support from loved ones and a strong social support network are crucial for individuals living with bipolar disorder. Family members and friends can provide emotional support, help with medication adherence, and assist in recognizing early warning signs of mood episodes. Support groups and online communities can also be valuable resources, allowing individuals to connect with others who share similar experiences and challenges.

Definition and types of bipolar disorders

Bipolar disorder is a mental health condition characterized by significant shifts in mood, energy levels, and activity patterns. It affects millions of people worldwide and can have a profound impact on their daily lives. Understanding the definition and different types of bipolar disorder is crucial for accurate diagnosis, appropriate treatment, and effective management of this complex condition.

Bipolar disorder, also known as manic, depressive illness, is marked by two distinct mood states: manic episodes and depressive episodes. During manic episodes, individuals experience an elevated or irritable mood, increased energy levels, racing thoughts, and impulsive behavior. They may feel invincible, engage in reckless activities, and have a decreased need for sleep. In contrast, depressive episodes involve persistent feelings of sadness, hopelessness, low energy, loss of interest in previously enjoyed activities, and difficulty concentrating. These mood swings can vary in duration, ranging from days to weeks or even months.

There are several types of bipolar disorder, each characterized by the severity and duration of manic and depressive episodes. Bipolar I disorder is the most severe form, involving full, blown manic episodes that can last for at least seven days or require hospitalization. Depressive episodes may also occur, lasting for a minimum of two weeks. Bipolar II disorder is characterized by recurring depressive episodes and hypomanic episodes, which are less severe than full manic episodes. Hypomanic episodes typically last for at least four days.

Cyclothymic disorder is another type of bipolar disorder, characterized by numerous periods of hypomanic symptoms and depressive symptoms that persist for at least two years in adults (one year in children and adolescents). However, the symptoms do not meet the full criteria for manic or depressive episodes. Cyclothymic disorder is often a milder form of bipolar disorder but can still significantly impact an individual's functioning and well, being.

In addition to these primary types, there are other specified and unspecified bipolar and related disorders. These include bipolar disorder due to another medical condition, such as a substance use disorder or a neurological disorder, as well as bipolar and related disorders induced by certain medications or substances. These categories are used when the bipolar symptoms are attributed to a specific cause and do not fit the criteria for the other established types of bipolar disorder.

It is worth noting that bipolar disorder can also present as rapid cycling, which refers to the occurrence of at least four mood episodes (manic, hypomanic, or depressive) within a year. Rapid cycling can make the management of bipolar disorder more challenging, as individuals experience more frequent and intense mood swings.

The exact causes of bipolar disorder are not fully understood, but researchers believe that a combination of genetic, biological, and environmental factors play a role in its development. Studies have shown that individuals with a family history of bipolar disorder are more likely to develop the condition themselves, suggesting a genetic predisposition. Biological factors, such as imbalances in neurotransmitters like serotonin and dopamine, may also contribute to the onset and progression of bipolar disorder. Environmental factors, including stressful life events, traumatic experiences, and substance abuse, can trigger or exacerbate episodes in susceptible individuals.

Accurate diagnosis of bipolar disorder requires a comprehensive evaluation by a qualified healthcare professional, typically a psychiatrist. The Diagnostic and Statistical Manual of Mental Disorders (DSM, 5) provides the criteria used for diagnosing bipolar disorder. It is crucial to differentiate bipolar disorder from other mental health conditions that share similar symptoms, such as major depressive disorder or borderline personality disorder, as the treatment approaches may vary.

Treatment for bipolar disorder usually involves a combination of medication, psychotherapy, and lifestyle adjustments. Mood stabilizers, such as lithium, valproate, or anticonvulsant medications, are commonly prescribed to help manage mood swings and prevent relapses.

The bipolar spectrum: from cyclothymia to bipolar I and II

Bipolar disorder is a complex mental health condition characterized by significant mood swings, ranging from manic highs to depressive lows. Within the realm of bipolar disorders, there exists a spectrum that encompasses various subtypes, each with its unique features and severity. Understanding the bipolar spectrum, from cyclothymia to bipolar I and II, is crucial for accurate diagnosis, appropriate treatment, and effective management of these conditions.

At one end of the bipolar spectrum lies cyclothymia, often considered a milder form of bipolar disorder. Individuals with cyclothymia experience recurrent periods of hypomanic symptoms and depressive symptoms that persist for at least two years in adults (one year in children and adolescents). However, these symptoms do not meet the full criteria for manic or depressive episodes seen in other bipolar disorders. Cyclothymic individuals may have periods of elevated mood, increased energy, and impulsivity, which are less intense than those seen in full, blown mania. Similarly, their depressive episodes may be less severe than those experienced by individuals with bipolar I or II disorder. Nonetheless, cyclothymia can still significantly impact an individual's functioning and well, being.

Moving further along the spectrum, we encounter bipolar II disorder. This subtype is characterized by recurring depressive episodes and hypomanic episodes. Hypomanic episodes, which are less severe than full, blown manic episodes, involve a distinct period of increased energy, elevated mood, and heightened productivity. Individuals experiencing hypomania may feel more confident, engage in goal, directed activities, and require less sleep. Unlike manic episodes seen in bipolar I disorder, hypomanic episodes do not result in severe impairment or require hospitalization. However, the presence of depressive episodes can make the overall impact of bipolar II disorder substantial. The depressive episodes in bipolar II disorder can be severe, characterized by persistent sadness, loss of interest, and feelings of hopelessness.

On the other end of the spectrum is bipolar I disorder, the most severe form of the condition. Bipolar I disorder involves full, blown manic episodes that last for at least seven days or require hospitalization. Manic episodes are marked by an intense euphoria or irritability, racing thoughts, inflated self, esteem, and impulsive behavior. Individuals in a manic state may engage in reckless activities, exhibit poor judgment, and experience a decreased need for sleep. The manic episodes in bipolar I disorder can be so severe that they lead to significant impairment in various aspects of life, including work, relationships, and personal well, being. Depressive episodes may also occur in bipolar I disorder, characterized by profound sadness, loss of interest, and feelings of worthlessness.

It is important to note that bipolar disorder can also present with mixed features, blurring the boundaries between mania and depression. Mixed episodes involve the simultaneous presence of manic and depressive symptoms, leading to a state of agitation, irritability, and heightened risk for impulsive actions. Individuals experiencing mixed episodes may feel overwhelmed, restless, and experience a rapid cycling between different mood states.

The bipolar spectrum also includes other specified and unspecified bipolar and related disorders. These categories are used when the symptoms of bipolar disorder are attributed to a specific cause and do not fit the criteria for the established types. For example, bipolar disorder due to another medical condition or substance, induced bipolar disorder may be diagnosed if the symptoms result from a medical condition or substance abuse.

Accurate diagnosis of bipolar disorder and its specific subtype requires a comprehensive evaluation by a qualified healthcare professional, typically a psychiatrist. The Diagnostic and Statistical Manual of Mental Disorders (DSM, 5) provides the criteria used for diagnosing bipolar disorders and helps guide treatment decisions.

Chapter Two

Symptoms and Diagnosis

Bipolar disorders are mental health conditions characterized by extreme mood swings, including periods of mania and depression. Recognizing the symptoms and obtaining an accurate diagnosis are crucial for individuals seeking treatment and support. Understanding the diverse range of symptoms associated with bipolar disorders and the diagnostic process can help improve outcomes for those affected by this complex condition.

The symptoms of bipolar disorders can vary widely, depending on the specific subtype and the current mood state. Manic episodes are characterized by an elevated mood or irritability, increased energy levels, racing thoughts, and a sense of grandiosity. Individuals in a manic state may exhibit impulsive behavior, engage in risky activities, and have a decreased need for sleep. They may also experience an inflated sense of self, esteem, talk excessively, and exhibit distractibility.

In contrast, depressive episodes involve persistent feelings of sadness, hopelessness, and low energy levels. Individuals experiencing depression may lose interest in activities they once enjoyed, have difficulty concentrating, and experience changes in appetite and sleep patterns. They may also contemplate self, harm or have thoughts of suicide. Depressive episodes can significantly impair functioning and negatively impact relationships, work, and overall well, being.

One of the challenges in diagnosing bipolar disorders is the variability of symptoms and the overlap with other mental health conditions. Bipolar disorders can be misdiagnosed as major depressive disorder or other mood disorders, leading to ineffective treatment. Accurate diagnosis requires a comprehensive psychiatric evaluation by a qualified healthcare professional, typically a psychiatrist.

The Diagnostic and Statistical Manual of Mental Disorders (DSM, 5) provides criteria that aid in the diagnosis of bipolar disorders. To meet the criteria for bipolar I disorder, individuals must have experienced at least one manic episode. Bipolar II disorder is diagnosed when individuals have had at least one hypomanic episode and one major depressive episode. Hypomanic episodes are less severe than full, blown manic episodes but still exhibit distinct changes in mood, energy levels, and behavior. Cyclothymic disorder, another subtype on the bipolar spectrum, involves numerous periods of hypomanic and depressive symptoms that persist for at least two years (one year in children and adolescents).

The diagnostic process typically involves a detailed assessment of an individual's symptoms, medical history, and family history of mental health conditions. Healthcare professionals may use standardized questionnaires and rating scales to gather information about the severity and duration of mood symptoms. They may also conduct interviews with the individual and their loved ones to gain a comprehensive understanding of the symptoms and their impact on daily life.

It is important to note that bipolar disorder can coexist with other mental health conditions, known as comorbidities. Conditions such as anxiety disorders, substance use disorders, and attention, deficit/hyperactivity disorder (ADHD) are commonly seen alongside bipolar disorders. Identifying and addressing these comorbidities is essential for providing comprehensive care and improving overall outcomes.

The accurate diagnosis of bipolar disorders goes beyond simply identifying the presence of manic and depressive episodes. Healthcare professionals also consider the frequency and duration of mood episodes, the level of impairment experienced, and any specific features such as rapid cycling or mixed features. The diagnostic process is an ongoing and dynamic process, as individuals may experience changes in symptoms over time.

In addition to the clinical assessment, clinicians may also utilize other tools, such as medical tests and imaging studies, to rule out potential medical conditions or substance, induced symptoms that may mimic bipolar disorders. This comprehensive evaluation helps ensure that the symptoms are not solely attributable to another medical condition or substance use.

Obtaining an accurate diagnosis is crucial as it guides treatment decisions and helps individuals access appropriate care and support. Early detection and intervention can lead to better outcomes and improved quality of life for those affected by bipolar disorders.

Manic episodes: signs, symptoms, and severity

Manic episodes are a key characteristic of bipolar disorders, representing a distinct period of intense and heightened mood. Understanding the signs, symptoms, and severity of manic episodes is crucial for accurately diagnosing and managing bipolar disorders. These episodes can significantly impact an individual's life and require appropriate treatment and support.

During a manic episode, individuals experience an abnormally elevated mood or extreme irritability that is distinctly different from their usual state. This elevated mood is one of the defining features of mania and sets it apart from other mood disorders. The signs and symptoms of a manic episode can vary in intensity and duration, but they generally share common characteristics.

One of the primary signs of a manic episode is a significantly increased energy level. Individuals may feel an extreme burst of energy and engage in activities more vigorously than usual. They may exhibit hyperactivity, restlessness, and have a constant need to keep busy. This surplus of energy often leads to a reduced need for sleep. Individuals in a manic state may feel rested even after just a few hours of sleep, or they may experience periods of insomnia.

Another hallmark symptom of a manic episode is racing thoughts. Individuals often experience a flood of ideas and have difficulty keeping their thoughts organized. Their mind may jump from one topic to another rapidly, making it challenging to concentrate or engage in focused activities. This can lead to distractibility and an inability to complete tasks.

Individuals in a manic state may exhibit increased talkativeness. They may talk rapidly and incessantly, often switching from one topic to another without pause. Their speech may become loud, pressured, and difficult to interrupt. This excessive verbal output is a prominent feature of a manic episode and can be noticeable to others.

One of the most noticeable symptoms of mania is an inflated sense of self, esteem or grandiosity. Individuals may believe they possess special abilities, talents, or powers. They may have an exaggerated belief in their importance, considering themselves to be superior to others. This grandiosity can lead to a sense of entitlement and an expectation of special treatment.

Impulsivity and reckless behavior are also common during a manic episode. Individuals may engage in activities that have high potential for negative consequences, such as excessive spending, risky sexual behavior, or substance abuse. They may make impulsive decisions without considering the long, term consequences or engaging in dangerous activities without regard for personal safety.

The severity of manic episodes can vary among individuals and even within the same individual over time. In some cases, the manic episode may be mild, with symptoms that are manageable and do not lead to significant impairment in daily functioning. However, in more severe cases, individuals may experience extreme and disruptive symptoms that require hospitalization or intensive treatment.

It is important to note that severe manic episodes can result in a loss of touch with reality, a condition known as psychosis. Psychotic symptoms may include hallucinations (perceiving things that are not actually present) or delusions (false beliefs that are not based in reality). These symptoms can further exacerbate the impact of a manic episode on an individual's life and necessitate immediate medical attention.

Diagnosing a manic episode involves a comprehensive psychiatric evaluation by a healthcare professional, typically a psychiatrist. The clinician will assess the presence and duration of symptoms, their impact on daily functioning, and any associated features such as rapid cycling or mixed features. The Diagnostic and Statistical Manual of Mental Disorders (DSM, 5) provides specific criteria for diagnosing manic episodes and bipolar disorders.

Treating manic episodes typically involves a combination of medications and psychotherapy. Mood stabilizers, such as lithium or anticonvulsant medications, are commonly prescribed to help manage the symptoms and stabilize mood. Antipsychotic medications may be utilized if psychotic symptoms are present.

Depressive episodes: signs, symptoms, and severity

Depressive episodes are a significant component of bipolar disorders, characterized by intense feelings of sadness, hopelessness, and a loss of interest in previously enjoyed activities. Understanding the signs, symptoms, and severity of depressive episodes is crucial for accurate diagnosis and effective management of bipolar disorders. These episodes can have a profound impact on individuals' lives, requiring appropriate treatment and support.

During a depressive episode, individuals experience persistent and pervasive feelings of sadness, emptiness, and low mood. These emotions are often disproportionate to the circumstances and can persist for an extended period. Depressive episodes are characterized by a cluster of symptoms that affect various aspects of an individual's life.

One of the core symptoms of a depressive episode is a persistent feeling of sadness or emptiness. Individuals may describe a sense of despair and find it challenging to experience pleasure or joy in activities they once enjoyed. They may withdraw from social interactions, lose interest in hobbies or work, and experience a general lack of motivation.

Depressive episodes often lead to a decrease in energy levels and increased fatigue. Individuals may feel physically and mentally drained, lacking the energy to engage in daily tasks. Even small activities may feel exhausting and overwhelming. The experience of fatigue can be debilitating and further contribute to the sense of hopelessness and despair.

Changes in appetite and weight are common symptoms of a depressive episode. Some individuals may experience a decrease in appetite and weight loss, while others may find comfort in food and experience an increase in appetite and subsequent weight gain. These changes are not related to intentional dietary modifications but are a result of the underlying depressive symptoms.

Sleep disturbances are also prevalent during depressive episodes. Individuals may experience insomnia, struggling to fall asleep or stay asleep throughout the night. Conversely, others may experience hypersomnia, finding it difficult to wake up in the morning and spending excessive amounts of time in bed. Sleep disturbances can exacerbate feelings of fatigue and contribute to the overall impact of depressive episodes on an individual's functioning.

Feelings of worthlessness, excessive guilt, and self, criticism are common cognitive symptoms experienced during depressive episodes. Individuals may have negative thoughts about themselves, their abilities, and their accomplishments. They may dwell on past failures or perceive themselves as burdens to others. These negative self, perceptions can intensify the feelings of sadness and hopelessness associated with depression.

Depressive episodes can also manifest with physical symptoms. Individuals may experience physical aches and pains, headaches, or digestive problems without any apparent medical cause. These physical symptoms often coexist with the psychological and emotional symptoms of depression, contributing to the overall burden of the episode.

The severity of depressive episodes can vary widely among individuals and within the same individual over time. In some cases, the depressive episode may be mild, with symptoms that do not significantly impair daily functioning. However, in more severe cases, individuals may experience intense and persistent symptoms that severely impact their ability to carry out routine activities or maintain relationships. Severe depressive episodes can be accompanied by thoughts of self, harm or suicide, requiring immediate attention and intervention.

Diagnosing a depressive episode as part of bipolar disorder involves a comprehensive psychiatric evaluation by a healthcare professional. The clinician will assess the presence and duration of symptoms, their impact on daily functioning, and any associated features such as rapid cycling or mixed features. The Diagnostic and Statistical Manual of Mental Disorders (DSM, 5) provides specific criteria for diagnosing depressive episodes and bipolar disorders.

Treatment for depressive episodes in bipolar disorders often involves a combination of medication and psychotherapy. Antidepressant medications may be prescribed to alleviate depressive symptoms. However, they are typically used with caution in bipolar disorders, as they can potentially trigger manic episodes.

Hypomanic episodes: distinguishing from mania

Hypomanic episodes are a distinctive feature of bipolar disorders, characterized by periods of elevated mood and increased energy. Understanding the differences between hypomania and full, blown mania is essential for accurate diagnosis and effective management of bipolar disorders. Distinguishing the characteristics of hypomanic episodes from manic episodes helps healthcare professionals develop appropriate treatment plans and support individuals experiencing these episodes.

Hypomania shares similarities with mania but differs in terms of severity, duration, and impact on daily functioning. While both hypomania and mania involve an elevated mood, hypomania is considered a less severe form of mood disturbance. During a hypomanic episode, individuals experience a distinct period of abnormally elevated or irritable mood, accompanied by increased energy and activity.

One key feature that distinguishes hypomania from mania is the absence of marked impairment in functioning. Unlike in manic episodes, individuals experiencing hypomania can generally continue with their daily activities and responsibilities without significant disruption. Although they may exhibit heightened productivity, increased sociability, and a sense of well, being, they can still maintain social and occupational functioning.

Another difference between hypomania and mania is the duration of the episode. Hypomanic episodes typically last for at least four consecutive days. In contrast, manic episodes extend beyond one week, often requiring hospitalization due to the severity of symptoms and impaired judgment. The shorter duration of hypomanic episodes contributes to the milder impact on an individual's life.

While hypomanic episodes are less severe than manic episodes, they share common symptoms. Individuals in a hypomanic state may exhibit increased energy, decreased need for sleep, and racing thoughts. They may engage in goal, directed activities, demonstrate high levels of productivity, and appear more sociable and talkative than usual. These symptoms reflect the heightened energy and increased motivation characteristic of hypomania.

During hypomanic episodes, individuals may experience an inflated sense of self, esteem or grandiosity. They may feel unusually confident, capable, and believe they possess special talents or abilities. This heightened self, perception can contribute to a sense of invincibility and increased risk, taking behavior. However, the impulsive actions associated with hypomania tend to be less extreme than those observed during manic episodes.

It is important to note that while hypomanic episodes do not typically cause significant impairment, they can still impact an individual's life in subtle ways. The changes in mood and behavior can strain relationships, disrupt sleep patterns, and influence decision, making. The impact of hypomania can also be cumulative, as multiple episodes over time can contribute to fluctuations in overall functioning and emotional stability.

Distinguishing between hypomanic and manic episodes is crucial for accurate diagnosis and appropriate treatment. The Diagnostic and Statistical Manual of Mental Disorders (DSM, 5) provides specific criteria for differentiating between these episodes. For a diagnosis of bipolar II disorder, individuals must have experienced at least one hypomanic episode and one major depressive episode. Bipolar I disorder, on the other hand, is characterized by the presence of at least one manic episode.

Treatment for hypomanic episodes often involves a combination of medication and psychotherapy. Mood stabilizers, such as lithium or anticonvulsant medications, are commonly prescribed to help regulate mood and prevent the escalation of hypomania into full, blown mania. Psychotherapy, such as cognitive, behavioral therapy (CBT), can be beneficial in helping individuals identify triggers, develop coping strategies, and manage the impact of hypomanic episodes on their lives.

Mixed episodes: combining manic and depressive symptoms

Mixed episodes are a unique and complex feature of bipolar disorders, characterized by the simultaneous presence of manic and depressive symptoms. Understanding mixed episodes is crucial for accurate diagnosis, appropriate treatment, and effective management of bipolar disorders. These episodes present unique challenges and require a comprehensive approach to address the diverse and often conflicting symptoms.

In typical bipolar disorder episodes, individuals experience distinct periods of either mania or depression. However, in a mixed episode, the symptoms of both manic and depressive states occur simultaneously, resulting in a tumultuous and intense emotional experience. This combination of symptoms creates a unique clinical picture and can be particularly challenging for individuals and their healthcare providers.

During a mixed episode, individuals may feel a mix of high energy and low mood, leading to a state of agitation and restlessness. They may experience rapid shifts in emotions, alternating between feelings of euphoria and sadness or irritability. The coexistence of manic and depressive symptoms can intensify emotional turmoil and lead to an overall sense of confusion and instability.

One of the hallmark features of a mixed episode is the presence of depressive symptoms alongside manic symptoms. Individuals may experience persistent feelings of sadness, hopelessness, and low self, esteem while also exhibiting signs of heightened energy, increased activity, and impulsivity. This combination can be distressing and result in an inner conflict, as the individual may feel torn between engaging in impulsive and potentially risky behaviors and experiencing a profound sense of sadness.

The presence of mixed episodes can further complicate the diagnosis and management of bipolar disorders. Healthcare professionals need to carefully assess the symptoms to differentiate a mixed episode from other conditions that may present with similar features, such as borderline personality disorder or rapid cycling bipolar disorder. A comprehensive evaluation of the individual's history, duration, and severity of symptoms is crucial for accurate diagnosis.

The Diagnostic and Statistical Manual of Mental Disorders (DSM, 5) provides specific criteria for diagnosing mixed episodes. To meet the criteria, an individual must experience a distinct period during which manic and depressive symptoms are present nearly every day for at least one week. These symptoms must cause significant impairment in functioning and are not attributable to the physiological effects of substance use or another medical condition.

Treating mixed episodes requires a comprehensive approach that addresses both manic and depressive symptoms. Medication management is often a key component of treatment. Mood stabilizers, such as lithium or anticonvulsant medications, may be prescribed to help regulate mood and mitigate both the manic and depressive aspects of the episode. In some cases, antipsychotic medications or antidepressants may be utilized to target specific symptoms.

Psychotherapy is another essential component of treatment for mixed episodes. Cognitive, behavioral therapy (CBT) can help individuals identify and challenge negative thought patterns, develop coping strategies, and enhance emotion regulation skills. Psychoeducation about bipolar disorders and strategies to manage symptoms during mixed episodes can empower individuals to take an active role in their treatment.

The management of mixed episodes also involves addressing immediate safety concerns. The risk of self, harm or suicide can be heightened during mixed episodes, given the intense emotional turmoil and conflicting symptoms. Healthcare professionals must assess the individual's risk and implement appropriate safety measures, including close monitoring, involvement of support systems, and ensuring access to crisis intervention resources.

Support from loved ones is crucial for individuals experiencing mixed episodes. Family members and friends can provide emotional support, assist with medication adherence, and help identify early warning signs of mixed episodes. They can also facilitate communication with healthcare providers and support the individual in adhering to treatment recommendations.

Chapter Three

Causes and Risk Factors

Bipolar disorders are complex mental health conditions characterized by extreme mood swings, including manic and depressive episodes. Understanding the causes and risk factors associated with bipolar disorders is essential for identifying vulnerable individuals, improving early detection, and developing effective treatment strategies. While the exact causes of bipolar disorders are not fully understood, researchers have identified several factors that contribute to their development.

Genetic Factors: Genetics plays a significant role in the development of bipolar disorders. Research has shown that individuals with a family history of bipolar disorders are more likely to develop the condition themselves. Studies involving twins have provided further evidence of the genetic basis of bipolar disorders, with higher concordance rates among identical twins compared to fraternal twins. Multiple genes are believed to be involved, although no single gene has been identified as the sole cause of bipolar disorders.

Neurochemical Imbalances: Imbalances in neurotransmitters, the chemical messengers in the brain, are thought to contribute to the development of bipolar disorders. Specifically, abnormalities in the regulation of serotonin, dopamine, and norepinephrine have been observed in individuals with bipolar disorders. These neurotransmitters play crucial roles in regulating mood, emotions, and cognitive processes. Imbalances in their levels and functioning can disrupt the stability of mood states, leading to the characteristic mood swings seen in bipolar disorders.

Biological Factors: Various biological factors have been implicated in the development of bipolar disorders. Structural and functional abnormalities in certain brain regions, such as the prefrontal cortex, amygdala, and hippocampus, have been observed in individuals with bipolar disorders. These brain regions are involved in emotion regulation, memory processing, and decision, making, all of which are disrupted during episodes of mania and depression. Hormonal imbalances, disrupted circadian rhythms, and immune system dysregulation have also been associated with bipolar disorders.

Environmental Triggers: While genetics and biological factors play significant roles, environmental factors can also trigger the onset of bipolar disorders or contribute to the severity of symptoms. Stressful life events, such as trauma, loss of a loved one, or significant life changes, can act as triggers for the first episode of mania or depression. Additionally, chronic stress, substance abuse, and disrupted sleep patterns can exacerbate symptoms and increase the risk of relapse in individuals already diagnosed with bipolar disorders.

Substance Abuse: Substance abuse is a significant risk factor for the development of bipolar disorders. Individuals who abuse drugs or alcohol are more likely to experience mood disturbances and episodes of mania or depression. Substance abuse can trigger the onset of bipolar episodes, worsen the course of the illness, and impair treatment outcomes. Additionally, substance abuse can complicate the diagnosis and management of bipolar disorders, making it challenging to differentiate between substance, induced mood symptoms and primary bipolar symptoms.

Childhood Trauma: Childhood trauma, including physical, sexual, or emotional abuse, neglect, or early loss of a parent, has been associated with an increased risk of developing bipolar disorders later in life. Adverse childhood experiences can have long, lasting effects on brain development, stress response systems, and emotional regulation, predisposing individuals to mental health conditions such as bipolar disorders.

Other Mental Health Conditions: Bipolar disorders often coexist with other mental health conditions. Conditions such as anxiety disorders, attention, deficit/hyperactivity disorder (ADHD), and borderline personality disorder are commonly observed in individuals with bipolar disorders. The presence of these comorbidities can complicate diagnosis and treatment, as symptoms may overlap or interact with bipolar symptoms, requiring a comprehensive approach to address multiple conditions.

Genetic factors and family history

Bipolar disorders are complex mental health conditions characterized by extreme mood swings, ranging from manic highs to depressive lows. While the exact causes of bipolar disorders are not fully understood, research has shown that genetic factors and family history play a significant role in their development. Understanding the influence of genetics on bipolar disorders can provide valuable insights into their etiology, improve early detection, and guide treatment strategies.

Genetic factors are believed to contribute significantly to the risk of developing bipolar disorders. Family, twin, and adoption studies have consistently demonstrated a higher prevalence of the disorder among close relatives of individuals with bipolar disorders. The heritability of bipolar disorders is estimated to be around 70, 80%, indicating a strong genetic influence.

Researchers have been investigating the specific genes involved in bipolar disorders, aiming to identify the genetic variants that increase susceptibility to the condition. Genome, wide association studies (GWAS) and candidate gene studies have identified several genes that may play a role in bipolar disorders, including ANK3, CACNA1C, and DGKH, among others. However, it is important to note that no single gene has been identified as the sole cause of bipolar disorders, as the condition is likely influenced by the interplay of multiple genes.

In addition to specific genes, researchers have also explored the impact of gene, environment interactions in bipolar disorders. Environmental factors, such as stress or substance abuse, can interact with genetic predispositions, potentially triggering the onset or exacerbating symptoms of bipolar disorders. For example, individuals with a genetic susceptibility to bipolar disorders may be more vulnerable to the effects of stressful life events, leading to the manifestation of the disorder. Similarly, substance abuse can interact with genetic factors, increasing the risk of developing bipolar disorders or worsening its course.

Family history is an important indicator of genetic risk for bipolar disorders. Individuals who have a first, degree relative, such as a parent or sibling, with bipolar disorders have a significantly higher risk of developing the condition themselves. The risk increases with the number of affected family members and is highest when both parents have bipolar disorders. However, it is important to note that having a family history of bipolar disorders does not guarantee that an individual will develop the condition. Many individuals with a family history of bipolar disorders do not develop the disorder, and conversely, some individuals without a family history can still develop bipolar disorders.

Understanding the genetic factors and family history of bipolar disorders has practical implications for clinical practice. Healthcare professionals often take into account a person's family history when making a diagnosis or assessing the risk of developing bipolar disorders. Individuals with a strong family history of bipolar disorders may be more closely monitored for early signs and symptoms, allowing for earlier intervention and treatment.

Genetic testing for bipolar disorders is not currently routine practice, as the genetic variants involved are not yet well, defined. However, advances in genetic research may lead to the development of genetic tests that can provide additional information about an individual's risk of developing bipolar disorders. Genetic testing may also help in personalizing treatment approaches by identifying specific genetic markers that can guide medication selection or predict treatment response.

It is important to note that while genetic factors and family history are significant contributors to the development of bipolar disorders, they are not the sole determining factors. Environmental influences, such as stressful life events, childhood trauma, or substance abuse, can also interact with genetic vulnerabilities to contribute to the onset and course of bipolar disorders.

Environmental factors and life events

Bipolar disorders are complex mental health conditions characterized by extreme mood swings, ranging from manic highs to depressive lows. While genetic factors play a significant role in their development, research has shown that environmental factors and life events also contribute to the onset and course of bipolar disorders. Understanding the influence of environmental factors can provide valuable insights into the disorder's etiology, inform prevention strategies, and guide treatment approaches.

Stressful Life Events: Stressful life events are often identified as triggers for the onset of bipolar episodes. Major life changes, such as loss of a loved one, relationship difficulties, financial stress, or significant work, related changes, can act as stressors that precipitate mood episodes in susceptible individuals. Stress disrupts the body's physiological response systems, including the hypothalamic, pituitary, adrenal (HPA) axis, leading to dysregulation of stress hormones and potentially triggering the manifestation of bipolar symptoms.

Childhood Trauma: Adverse childhood experiences, including physical, sexual, or emotional abuse, neglect, or early loss of a parent, have been associated with an increased risk of developing bipolar disorders later in life. Childhood trauma can have long, lasting effects on brain development, stress response systems, and emotional regulation, making individuals more susceptible to mental health conditions such as bipolar disorders. Traumatic experiences can disrupt the normal functioning of neurotransmitters and impact brain regions involved in mood regulation.

Substance Abuse: Substance abuse, including alcohol and illicit drug use, is a significant environmental factor that can interact with genetic vulnerabilities to increase the risk of bipolar disorders. Substance abuse can act as a trigger for the onset of mood episodes or exacerbate existing symptoms. Individuals with bipolar disorders are more likely to engage in substance abuse as a means of self, medicating or managing the extreme mood swings associated with the condition. Substance abuse can also complicate the diagnosis and treatment of bipolar disorders, making it challenging to differentiate between substance, induced symptoms and primary bipolar symptoms.

Sleep Disturbances: Disruptions in sleep patterns, such as irregular sleep schedules, chronic sleep deprivation, or disturbances in circadian rhythms, can contribute to the onset and exacerbation of bipolar episodes. Sleep disturbances have been identified as potential prodromal symptoms of bipolar disorders, indicating an increased vulnerability to mood episodes.

Sleep deprivation can disrupt the balance of neurotransmitters, impair cognitive functioning, and contribute to mood dysregulation.

Social Support: Social support and interpersonal relationships play a crucial role in the management of bipolar disorders. Positive social support systems, including stable and nurturing relationships, can provide emotional validation, assistance with coping strategies, and practical help during difficult times. On the other hand, a lack of social support or strained relationships can increase the risk of mood episodes and hinder recovery. Stressful or dysfunctional family environments can contribute to increased symptom severity and decreased treatment adherence.

Parenting Style: Parenting practices and family dynamics can influence the development and course of bipolar disorders, especially during childhood and adolescence. Studies have suggested that parenting styles characterized by high levels of criticism, overinvolvement, or neglect may contribute to the development of bipolar disorders in vulnerable individuals. Negative family interactions and high levels of expressed emotion can exacerbate stress and trigger mood episodes.

Seasonal Changes: Some individuals with bipolar disorders experience seasonal patterns, with mood episodes occurring during specific times of the year. Seasonal affective disorder (SAD), a subtype of depression associated with changes in light exposure during the winter months, can coexist with bipolar disorders. The disrupted circadian rhythms and reduced exposure to natural light during certain seasons can contribute to mood instability and trigger depressive or manic episodes.

Brain chemistry and neurobiological factors

Bipolar disorders are complex mental health conditions characterized by extreme mood swings, including manic highs and depressive lows. While genetic and environmental factors play significant roles in the development of bipolar disorders, research has also shed light on the crucial role of brain chemistry and neurobiological factors in the etiology and manifestation of the disorder. Understanding the underlying neurobiological mechanisms can provide valuable insights into the condition, guide treatment strategies, and inform future research endeavors.

Neurotransmitters: Neurotransmitters are chemical messengers that facilitate communication between neurons in the brain. Abnormalities in neurotransmitter systems have been implicated in bipolar disorders. Serotonin, dopamine, and norepinephrine are the key neurotransmitters involved in mood regulation. Fluctuations in the levels and functioning of these neurotransmitters can disrupt the delicate balance between excitatory and inhibitory processes, contributing to the mood swings observed in bipolar disorders. For instance, increased dopamine activity during manic episodes is associated with heightened energy, euphoria, and increased goal, directed behavior.

Neuroendocrine System: The neuroendocrine system, including the hypothalamic, pituitary, adrenal (HPA) axis, plays a crucial role in regulating the body's response to stress. Dysregulation of the HPA axis has been observed in individuals with bipolar disorders. Chronic stress, a known risk factor for bipolar disorders, can lead to alterations in the HPA axis, resulting in increased cortisol levels and disrupted stress response. Dysregulation of the HPA axis can contribute to mood dysregulation, cognitive impairment, and increased vulnerability to mood episodes.

Circadian Rhythms: The circadian rhythms, which regulate the sleep, wake cycle and other physiological processes, are disrupted in individuals with bipolar disorders. Sleep disturbances, including insomnia or hypersomnia, are common symptoms of both depressive and manic episodes. Disruptions in the timing and quality of sleep can further contribute to mood instability and trigger mood episodes. Disturbed circadian rhythms, involving abnormalities in melatonin secretion and clock genes, may play a role in the regulation of mood and the manifestation of bipolar disorders.

Neuroplasticity: Neuroplasticity refers to the brain's ability to adapt and change in response to experiences and environmental stimuli. Altered neuroplasticity has been observed in individuals with bipolar disorders. Structural and functional abnormalities in brain regions involved in emotion regulation, including the prefrontal cortex, amygdala, and hippocampus, have been found in individuals with bipolar disorders. These abnormalities can disrupt the neural circuits responsible for mood regulation, leading to the characteristic mood swings observed in bipolar disorders.

Glutamate and GABA: Glutamate and gamma, aminobutyric acid (GABA) are the primary excitatory and inhibitory neurotransmitters in the brain, respectively. Imbalances in the levels and functioning of glutamate and GABA have been implicated in bipolar disorders. Reduced GABA levels and increased glutamate activity have been observed during manic episodes. These imbalances can contribute to hyperexcitability and dysregulation of neural networks, leading to the characteristic manic symptoms. Conversely, decreased glutamate activity and disrupted GABAergic inhibition have been associated with depressive symptoms.

Ion Channels and Calcium Signaling: Ion channels, such as voltage, gated calcium channels, are critical for maintaining neuronal excitability and regulating neurotransmitter release. Dysregulation of ion channels and calcium signaling has been implicated in bipolar disorders. Altered calcium signaling can disrupt neurotransmitter release and impair synaptic functioning. Dysfunction in ion channels can lead to aberrant neuronal firing patterns and contribute to the mood instability observed in bipolar disorders.

Chapter Four

Diagnosis and Assessment

Accurate diagnosis and assessment are crucial for effectively managing bipolar disorders. The complex nature of these conditions, characterized by distinct episodes of mania and depression, requires a comprehensive evaluation to differentiate bipolar disorders from other mental health conditions. Diagnostic criteria, clinical interviews, and assessment tools play essential roles in the diagnostic process, helping healthcare professionals make informed decisions regarding treatment and support.

Diagnostic Criteria: The Diagnostic and Statistical Manual of Mental Disorders (DSM, 5) provides diagnostic criteria for bipolar disorders. According to the DSM, 5, to receive a diagnosis of bipolar I disorder, an individual must have experienced at least one manic episode. A manic episode is characterized by a distinct period of elevated, expansive, or irritable mood, accompanied by increased energy and goal, directed activity. For a diagnosis of bipolar II disorder, at least one hypomanic episode and one major depressive episode are required. Hypomanic episodes involve similar symptoms as manic episodes but are of shorter duration and do not cause severe impairment in functioning.

Clinical Interviews: Clinical interviews are an integral part of the diagnostic process for bipolar disorders. A thorough assessment is conducted by a mental health professional, typically a psychiatrist or psychologist, to gather information about the individual's medical history, family history, and current symptoms. The clinician will ask specific questions to assess the presence of manic, hypomanic, or depressive symptoms, their duration and severity, and the impact on daily functioning. Clinical interviews also allow for the exploration of potential co, occurring mental health conditions or substance abuse, which can complicate the diagnosis and treatment of bipolar disorders.

Mood Symptom Questionnaires: Various self, report questionnaires and rating scales are used to assess mood symptoms and their severity in individuals suspected of having bipolar disorders. These measures, such as the Mood Disorder Questionnaire (MDQ) or the Young Mania Rating Scale (YMRS), help quantify the presence and intensity of manic or hypomanic symptoms. Similarly, depression, specific scales like the Hamilton Depression Rating Scale (HDRS) or the Beck Depression Inventory (BDI) assist in assessing the severity of depressive symptoms. These measures serve as adjuncts to clinical interviews, providing additional information to support the diagnostic process.

Structured Clinical Interviews: Structured clinical interviews, such as the Structured Clinical Interview for DSM, 5 (SCID), are standardized assessment tools designed to systematically evaluate psychiatric disorders. These interviews provide a structured framework for assessing symptoms and applying diagnostic criteria. The SCID is widely used in research settings and can assist clinicians in making accurate diagnoses by ensuring a comprehensive and consistent evaluation of symptoms.

Longitudinal Assessment: Bipolar disorders are characterized by episodic fluctuations in mood. Therefore, a longitudinal assessment is essential for an accurate diagnosis. A single evaluation may not capture the full range of symptoms and mood episodes experienced by individuals with bipolar disorders. Tracking the individual's mood over time, gathering information from multiple sources (such as family members or close friends), and considering the presence of symptoms across different contexts can aid in identifying the pattern and severity of mood episodes.

Differential Diagnosis: Differential diagnosis involves distinguishing bipolar disorders from other mental health conditions that may present with similar symptoms. Conditions such as major depressive disorder, borderline personality disorder, attention, deficit/hyperactivity disorder (ADHD), or substance, induced mood disorders can exhibit overlapping symptoms with bipolar disorders. Careful consideration of the specific diagnostic criteria, the temporal pattern of symptoms, and the presence of manic or hypomanic episodes is crucial in differentiating bipolar disorders from other conditions.

Diagnostic criteria and the DSM

,

5

Accurate diagnosis is a fundamental step in effectively managing bipolar disorders. The Diagnostic and Statistical Manual of Mental Disorders (DSM, 5) provides a comprehensive framework for diagnosing mental health conditions, including bipolar disorders. Understanding the diagnostic criteria outlined in the DSM, 5 is essential for healthcare professionals to assess symptoms, make appropriate diagnoses, and guide treatment decisions in individuals with bipolar disorders.

The DSM, 5 provides specific criteria for diagnosing different types of bipolar disorders, including bipolar I disorder, bipolar II disorder, and cyclothymic disorder. The primary distinction between these disorders lies in the presence and duration of manic, hypomanic, and depressive episodes.

Bipolar I Disorder: Bipolar I disorder is characterized by the presence of at least one manic episode, which may be preceded or followed by hypomanic or depressive episodes. A manic episode is defined as a distinct period of abnormally elevated, expansive, or irritable mood, lasting for at least one week. During this period, individuals may experience increased energy, inflated self, esteem, decreased need for sleep, racing thoughts, excessive talking, and engaging in activities with high potential for painful consequences. The episode is severe enough to cause significant impairment in social, occupational, or other important areas of functioning.

Bipolar II Disorder: Bipolar II disorder involves at least one major depressive episode and at least one hypomanic episode. A major depressive episode is characterized by a two, week period of depressed mood or loss of interest or pleasure in activities. The symptoms must be present for most of the day, nearly every day, and significantly impair social, occupational, or other important areas of functioning. A hypomanic episode, in contrast to a full manic episode, is characterized by a distinct period of abnormally elevated or irritable mood lasting for at least four consecutive days. Hypomanic episodes are associated with increased energy, heightened productivity, and a sense of well, being but do not cause significant impairment.

Cyclothymic Disorder: Cyclothymic disorder involves chronic fluctuations in mood, with numerous periods of hypomanic symptoms and depressive symptoms over a two, year period. However, the symptoms do not meet the full criteria for a hypomanic episode or a major depressive episode. The mood swings in cyclothymic disorder are less severe and less disruptive to daily functioning compared to bipolar I or II disorders.

In addition to meeting the specific diagnostic criteria for each disorder, it is important to consider the temporal pattern and duration of symptoms. The DSM, 5 emphasizes the need to rule out other potential causes of mood disturbances, such as substance abuse, medical conditions, or the effects of medications.

While the DSM, 5 provides standardized criteria for diagnosing bipolar disorders, it also recognizes the dimensional nature of these conditions. Bipolar disorders exist along a spectrum, with varying degrees of severity and symptom expression. The DSM, 5 introduced a "specifier" system that allows clinicians to specify certain features of bipolar disorders, such as the presence of rapid cycling (four or more mood episodes in a year) or mixed features (the presence of manic or hypomanic symptoms during a major depressive episode).

It is important to note that the DSM, 5 is not without limitations. The diagnostic criteria are based on a consensus of expert opinions and research findings but may not capture the full complexity of bipolar disorders in every individual. Additionally, cultural factors and individual variations can influence the manifestation and interpretation of symptoms. Therefore, clinical judgment and consideration of the individual's unique presentation are crucial in making accurate diagnoses.

The role of mental health professionals

Bipolar disorders are complex mental health conditions characterized by extreme mood swings, including manic highs and depressive lows. The diagnosis, treatment, and management of bipolar disorders require the expertise of mental health professionals who play a vital role in providing comprehensive care to individuals affected by these conditions. Mental health professionals, such as psychiatrists, psychologists, and psychiatric nurses, contribute their specialized knowledge and skills to assess, diagnose, and support individuals with bipolar disorders throughout their treatment journey.

Assessment and Diagnosis: Mental health professionals are responsible for conducting thorough assessments to evaluate the presence and severity of bipolar symptoms. Through clinical interviews, psychological evaluations, and the utilization of standardized assessment tools, mental health professionals gather information about the individual's medical history, family history, and current symptoms. They explore the presence of manic, hypomanic, and depressive episodes, as well as the impact of these episodes on the individual's functioning. Accurate assessment and diagnosis are crucial for developing appropriate treatment plans and interventions.

Treatment Planning: Mental health professionals play a central role in developing individualized treatment plans for individuals with bipolar disorders. Based on the assessment findings, they collaborate with the individual to create a comprehensive treatment approach that addresses the unique needs and challenges associated with bipolar disorders. Treatment plans often involve a combination of medication management, psychotherapy, and lifestyle interventions. Mental health professionals take into account the individual's preferences, goals, and potential barriers to treatment adherence when formulating these plans.

Medication Management: Psychopharmacological treatment is a cornerstone of bipolar disorder management. Psychiatrists, who are medical doctors specializing in mental health, are primarily responsible for prescribing and monitoring medications to stabilize mood and manage symptoms. They assess the individual's specific symptom profile, medical history, and potential medication interactions to determine the most appropriate medication regimen. Regular follow, up appointments allow psychiatrists to monitor medication efficacy, adjust dosages if necessary, and manage any side effects. Close collaboration between mental health professionals and individuals is essential for successful medication management.

Psychotherapy: Psychotherapy, such as cognitive, behavioral therapy (CBT), interpersonal therapy (IPT), or family, focused therapy (FFT), is an integral component of bipolar disorder treatment. Psychologists, counselors, and social workers are trained in various psychotherapeutic approaches and work collaboratively with individuals to address the emotional, cognitive, and behavioral aspects of bipolar disorders. Psychotherapy aims to enhance coping skills, manage stress, regulate emotions, and prevent relapse. Mental health professionals provide a safe and supportive environment for individuals to explore their thoughts, emotions, and behaviors related to bipolar disorders.

Psychoeducation: Mental health professionals play a critical role in providing psychoeducation to individuals with bipolar disorders and their families. They offer information about the nature of bipolar disorders, including its causes, symptoms, and treatment options. Psychoeducation helps individuals understand their condition, recognize early warning signs of mood episodes, and learn strategies to manage symptoms effectively. Mental health professionals also educate families about bipolar disorders to foster a supportive environment and enhance family coping skills.

Crisis Intervention: Bipolar disorders can involve periods of acute crisis, such as severe depressive or manic episodes. Mental health professionals are trained in crisis intervention techniques to provide immediate support and assistance during these challenging times. They assess the individual's safety, develop crisis plans, and help facilitate hospitalization if necessary. Crisis intervention helps stabilize the individual and prevents harm or further exacerbation of symptoms.

Assessing severity and functional impairment

Bipolar disorders are complex mental health conditions characterized by extreme mood swings, ranging from manic highs to depressive lows. Assessing the severity of symptoms and functional impairment is crucial for understanding the impact of bipolar disorders on an individual's daily life and guiding treatment decisions. Mental health professionals utilize various assessment measures and tools to evaluate the severity of symptoms and the extent to which they interfere with an individual's functioning.

Symptom Severity Assessment: To assess the severity of symptoms in bipolar disorders, mental health professionals employ standardized rating scales and questionnaires. These tools help quantify the intensity and frequency of manic, hypomanic, and depressive symptoms experienced by individuals. Rating scales such as the Young Mania Rating Scale (YMRS) and the Hamilton Depression Rating Scale (HDRS) provide a systematic and objective means of evaluating symptom severity. By utilizing these scales, mental health professionals can track changes in symptomatology over time and assess the effectiveness of interventions.

Mood Monitoring: Regular mood monitoring is an important component of assessing severity in bipolar disorders. Individuals are encouraged to track their mood fluctuations, energy levels, and other relevant symptoms using daily mood charts or smartphone applications. This self, reporting method allows mental health professionals to gain insights into the pattern, duration, and severity of mood episodes. Mood monitoring provides a comprehensive picture of the individual's symptomatology and aids in identifying early warning signs of impending mood shifts.

Impairment Assessment: In addition to symptom severity, mental health professionals assess the functional impairment caused by bipolar disorders. Functional impairment refers to the difficulties individuals face in various domains of life, such as work, relationships, and self, care, due to their symptoms. Structured interviews and self, report measures, such as the

Functioning Assessment Short Test (FAST) or the Sheehan Disability Scale (SDS), are used to evaluate the impact of bipolar disorders on an individual's ability to carry out daily activities. This assessment helps identify areas of functioning that are most affected and guides treatment planning accordingly.

Social and Occupational Assessment: Assessing social and occupational functioning is essential in determining the impact of bipolar disorders on an individual's relationships and work life. Mental health professionals evaluate the quality of interpersonal relationships, social support systems, and the individual's ability to engage in social activities. They also assess occupational functioning, including job performance, productivity, and the ability to maintain employment. By understanding the challenges individuals face in these domains, mental health professionals can provide targeted interventions and support to improve social and occupational outcomes.

Cognitive Assessment: Cognitive impairment is a common feature of bipolar disorders and can significantly impact an individual's functioning. Mental health professionals may conduct cognitive assessments to evaluate various cognitive domains, such as attention, memory, executive functioning, and processing speed. This assessment helps identify cognitive strengths and weaknesses, guiding the development of cognitive strategies and accommodations to enhance overall functioning. Cognitive impairment assessment also assists in differentiating bipolar disorders from other cognitive disorders or neurocognitive deficits.

Quality of Life Assessment: Assessing the overall quality of life is important in understanding the holistic impact of bipolar disorders on individuals. Mental health professionals utilize measures such as the Quality of Life Enjoyment and Satisfaction Questionnaire (Q, LES, Q) or the World Health Organization Quality of Life (WHOQOL) scale to evaluate an individual's subjective well, being, satisfaction with life, and overall functioning in various life domains. This assessment provides valuable information about the individual's subjective experience, treatment outcomes, and areas that require additional support.

Chapter Five

Treatment Options

Bipolar disorders are complex mental health conditions characterized by extreme mood swings, including manic highs and depressive lows. Effective treatment approaches aim to stabilize mood, manage symptoms, and improve overall functioning. The treatment of bipolar disorders typically involves a combination of pharmacotherapy, psychotherapy, and lifestyle interventions. Tailoring treatment to the individual's specific needs and preferences is essential for successful management of bipolar disorders.

Pharmacotherapy: Medications play a central role in the treatment of bipolar disorders, particularly in stabilizing mood and preventing mood episodes. Mood stabilizers, such as lithium, are commonly prescribed to manage and prevent manic and depressive episodes. Anticonvulsant medications, such as valproate or lamotrigine, may also be used as mood stabilizers. Atypical antipsychotics, such as olanzapine or quetiapine, can be effective in managing acute manic or mixed episodes. Antidepressants may be prescribed cautiously in combination with mood stabilizers to manage depressive symptoms. The choice of medication depends on various factors, including the individual's symptom profile, medical history, and treatment response.

Psychotherapy: Psychotherapy is an essential component of bipolar disorder treatment. Various approaches can be effective, including cognitive, behavioral therapy (CBT), interpersonal therapy (IPT), and family, focused therapy (FFT). CBT aims to identify and modify negative thought patterns and behaviors, helping individuals develop coping strategies and manage stressors. IPT focuses on improving interpersonal relationships and resolving conflicts that may contribute to mood episodes. FFT involves working with the individual and their family members to enhance communication, reduce stress, and promote adherence to treatment. Psychotherapy provides individuals with the tools and support necessary to manage their symptoms, regulate emotions, and improve overall well, being.

Lifestyle Interventions: Adopting a healthy lifestyle is important in managing bipolar disorders. Regular exercise, adequate sleep, and a balanced diet contribute to overall well, being and can help stabilize mood. Individuals with bipolar disorders should aim for consistent sleep patterns and practice good sleep hygiene. Avoiding alcohol and illicit substances is crucial, as substance abuse can worsen symptoms and interfere with treatment effectiveness. Stress reduction techniques, such as mindfulness meditation or relaxation exercises, can also be beneficial in managing stress and preventing mood episodes.

Psychoeducation: Psychoeducation is a vital component of bipolar disorder treatment. Providing individuals and their families with information about the condition, its symptoms, and available treatment options helps improve understanding and coping skills. Psychoeducation sessions can cover topics such as recognizing early warning signs of mood episodes, adhering to medication regimens, managing stress, and developing support systems. Educating family members and close friends about bipolar disorders enhances their ability to provide support and reduces stigma associated with the condition.

Support Groups: Support groups offer individuals with bipolar disorders an opportunity to connect with others who share similar experiences.

Peer support can be invaluable in reducing feelings of isolation, providing validation, and offering practical advice. Support groups can be in, person or online and may be facilitated by mental health professionals or led by individuals who have successfully managed their own bipolar disorders. Being part of a support group fosters a sense of community and encourages individuals to actively engage in their treatment.

Hospitalization and Crisis Intervention: In severe cases, hospitalization may be necessary to stabilize individuals experiencing acute manic or depressive episodes. Hospitalization provides a controlled environment where individuals can receive intensive treatment, including medication adjustments, therapy, and safety monitoring. Crisis intervention services, including helplines or crisis response teams, offer immediate support and assistance during periods of acute crisis. These services help ensure the safety of individuals at risk and connect them with appropriate care.

Collaborative Care: Collaborative care involves coordination among healthcare professionals involved in the treatment of bipolar disorders.

Psychotherapy: cognitive

,

behavioral therapy, family

,

focused therapy, and interpersonal and social rhythm therapy

Psychotherapy plays a vital role in the treatment of bipolar disorders, complementing medication management and addressing the psychological and social aspects of the condition. Several evidence, based psychotherapeutic approaches have been developed to specifically target the unique challenges faced by individuals with bipolar disorders. Cognitive, Behavioral Therapy (CBT), Family, Focused Therapy (FFT), and Interpersonal and Social Rhythm Therapy (IPSRT) are three prominent therapies that have shown effectiveness in managing symptoms, improving functioning, and preventing relapse in individuals with bipolar disorders.

Cognitive, Behavioral Therapy (CBT): CBT is a widely used therapeutic approach that focuses on identifying and modifying negative thought patterns and behaviors. In the context of bipolar disorders, CBT aims to help individuals recognize and challenge distorted beliefs and cognitive biases associated with mood episodes. It helps individuals develop coping strategies to manage stressors, regulate emotions, and prevent relapse. CBT also emphasizes psychoeducation about bipolar disorders, assisting individuals in understanding their condition, recognizing triggers, and developing effective problem, solving skills. By targeting maladaptive thoughts and behaviors, CBT empowers individuals to take an active role in managing their symptoms and improving their quality of life.

Family, Focused Therapy (FFT): Family, Focused Therapy recognizes the impact of family dynamics on the course and management of bipolar disorders. It involves working with the individual diagnosed with bipolar disorder and their family members to enhance communication, reduce conflict, and improve problem, solving skills. FFT provides psychoeducation about bipolar disorders to family members, helping them understand the nature of the condition and its impact on the individual's functioning. By improving family support and reducing family stress, FFT aims to enhance treatment adherence and prevent relapse. The therapy also focuses on building strategies for early detection of mood shifts and managing them effectively as a family unit. Through increased understanding and improved communication, FFT creates a supportive environment that aids in the long, term management of bipolar disorders.

Interpersonal and Social Rhythm Therapy (IPSRT): IPSRT recognizes the importance of maintaining regular daily routines, social relationships, and sleep, wake cycles in the management of bipolar disorders. The therapy focuses on stabilizing individuals' daily routines and social rhythms to promote stability in mood. IPSRT helps individuals identify and manage life events and interpersonal conflicts that can disrupt their routines and trigger mood episodes. By addressing social and interpersonal issues, IPSRT aims to improve social functioning and reduce the risk of relapse. Additionally, the therapy incorporates elements of psychoeducation, teaching individuals about the relationship between circadian rhythms, sleep, and mood regulation. IPSRT provides individuals with practical strategies to maintain regular routines and manage sleep disturbances, fostering stability and enhancing overall well, being.

These psychotherapeutic approaches are often integrated into the overall treatment plan for bipolar disorders, alongside medication management and lifestyle interventions. Each therapy has unique strategies and techniques tailored to address specific aspects of bipolar disorders, but they share common goals of symptom management, relapse prevention, and improved functioning.

It is important to note that these therapies are typically delivered by trained mental health professionals, such as psychologists, social workers, or psychiatrists, who specialize in treating bipolar disorders. Therapeutic sessions are conducted in a structured and collaborative manner, involving active participation from both the individual and the therapist.

Evidence supporting the effectiveness of these therapies has been established through research studies. Multiple randomized controlled trials have demonstrated their efficacy in reducing symptom severity, decreasing relapse rates, and improving overall functioning in individuals with bipolar disorders. Moreover, these therapies can be adapted to different phases of the disorder, such as acute episodes, maintenance, or early intervention, to meet the specific needs of the individual at each stage.

Medications: mood stabilizers, antipsychotics, and antidepressants

Medication management plays a crucial role in the treatment of bipolar disorders, helping to stabilize mood, manage symptoms, and prevent relapse. Several classes of medications have been shown to be effective in addressing the manic and depressive episodes associated with bipolar disorders. Mood stabilizers, antipsychotics, and antidepressants are commonly prescribed medications that aim to balance brain chemistry and regulate mood in individuals with bipolar disorders.

Mood Stabilizers: Mood stabilizers are the cornerstone of pharmacotherapy for bipolar disorders. Lithium, a naturally occurring element, is one of the most commonly prescribed mood stabilizers. It is effective in reducing the frequency and severity of manic and depressive episodes. Lithium works by modulating neurotransmitter activity, particularly norepinephrine and serotonin, which are involved in mood regulation. Other mood stabilizers, such as valproate (valproic acid) and lamotrigine, are also used to manage bipolar disorders. Valproate is effective in treating manic episodes, while lamotrigine is more commonly prescribed for depressive episodes. Mood stabilizers help prevent mood swings and maintain long, term stability, reducing the risk of relapse.

Antipsychotics: Antipsychotic medications are used to manage acute manic or mixed episodes in bipolar disorders. They are effective in reducing the severity of manic symptoms, such as agitation, irritability, and psychosis. Atypical antipsychotics, such as quetiapine, olanzapine, and risperidone, are commonly prescribed in the treatment of bipolar disorders. These medications target the dopamine and serotonin neurotransmitter systems, helping to regulate mood and decrease excessive excitability in the brain. Antipsychotics can be used as monotherapy for acute episodes or in combination with mood stabilizers for long, term maintenance.

Antidepressants: Antidepressant medications are cautiously used in the treatment of bipolar disorders, primarily to address depressive symptoms. However, their use requires careful consideration due to the potential risk of triggering manic or hypomanic episodes. Antidepressants are typically prescribed in combination with mood stabilizers to minimize this risk. Selective serotonin reuptake inhibitors (SSRIs), such as fluoxetine or sertraline, are commonly used as they have a lower risk of inducing mania compared to other classes of antidepressants. Antidepressants can help alleviate depressive symptoms, improve mood, and enhance overall functioning in individuals with bipolar disorders.

It is important to note that medication management for bipolar disorders should be individualized based on the specific symptoms, treatment response, and potential side effects. Close collaboration between the prescribing healthcare professional and the individual is essential to monitor the effectiveness and tolerability of the medications.

Regular follow, up appointments are necessary to assess the individual's response to medication, adjust dosages if needed, and manage any side effects. It may take time to find the right medication or combination of medications that work best for each individual. Medications should be taken as prescribed and not abruptly discontinued, as sudden discontinuation can lead to relapse or withdrawal symptoms.

While medications are a key component of bipolar disorder treatment, they are most effective when combined with other treatment modalities, such as psychotherapy and lifestyle interventions. Integrated treatment approaches provide a comprehensive approach to managing bipolar disorders and addressing the psychological, social, and lifestyle aspects of the condition.

It is important to be aware that all medications carry potential side effects. Common side effects of mood stabilizers and antipsychotics include weight gain, sedation, tremors, and gastrointestinal disturbances. Antidepressants may also have side effects such as sexual dysfunction, nausea, or changes in sleep patterns.

Electroconvulsive therapy and other brain stimulation techniques

In the treatment of bipolar disorders, medications and psychotherapy are the primary modalities used. However, in cases where these approaches do not yield satisfactory results, or when urgent intervention is needed, brain stimulation techniques may be considered. Electroconvulsive therapy (ECT) is the most well, known and established form of brain stimulation therapy, while other emerging techniques, such as transcranial magnetic stimulation (TMS) and vagus nerve stimulation (VNS), show promise in the management of bipolar disorders.

Electroconvulsive Therapy (ECT): ECT involves the controlled administration of electric currents to the brain to induce a therapeutic seizure. While the precise mechanism of action is not fully understood, ECT is believed to modify the neurotransmitter levels and the communication between brain regions, resulting in mood stabilization. ECT is primarily used in severe cases of bipolar disorder, particularly when individuals do not respond to or cannot tolerate medications. It is effective in treating acute manic, depressive, or mixed episodes, as well as in preventing relapse. ECT is generally administered under anesthesia and involves a series of treatments over a few weeks. Side effects, such as temporary memory loss and confusion, are typically short, term and can be managed with proper monitoring and care.

Transcranial Magnetic Stimulation (TMS): TMS is a non, invasive brain stimulation technique that uses magnetic fields to stimulate specific regions of the brain. It is primarily used for the treatment of depressive episodes in bipolar disorders, especially when antidepressant medications are ineffective or not well, tolerated. TMS targets the prefrontal cortex, an area of the brain associated with mood regulation. The magnetic pulses stimulate neural activity, promoting the release of neurotransmitters involved in mood regulation. TMS is typically administered in an outpatient setting, with several sessions over a few weeks. It is well, tolerated and does not require anesthesia. Side effects are generally mild and include scalp discomfort or headaches.

Vagus Nerve Stimulation (VNS): VNS involves the implantation of a device that delivers electrical impulses to the vagus nerve, a major nerve that connects the brain to various organs in the body. VNS is thought to modulate neural activity and influence neurotransmitter levels, contributing to mood stabilization. While VNS is primarily used in the treatment of treatment, resistant depression, there is growing evidence supporting its potential benefits in bipolar disorders. It may help reduce the frequency and severity of mood episodes and improve overall functioning. VNS requires surgical implantation of the device, which is typically well, tolerated.

Side effects, such as hoarseness, cough, or neck discomfort, can usually be managed with adjustments to the device settings.

Deep Brain Stimulation (DBS): DBS is a more invasive brain stimulation technique that involves the surgical placement of electrodes in specific brain regions. These electrodes deliver electrical impulses to modulate neural activity and improve mood regulation. While DBS is still in the experimental stage for bipolar disorders, it has shown potential in targeting specific brain regions implicated in mood dysregulation. DBS is considered a last resort treatment for severe and treatment, resistant cases of bipolar disorders, as it involves surgical intervention and carries potential risks and complications. Ongoing research is exploring its safety and efficacy in the management of bipolar disorders.

Brain stimulation techniques, including ECT, TMS, VNS, and DBS, offer additional options for individuals with bipolar disorders who do not respond adequately to conventional treatments or who require urgent intervention. These techniques are generally reserved for severe or treatment, resistant cases under the guidance of specialized healthcare professionals.

Chapter Six

Managing Bipolar Disorder

Managing Bipolar Disorder: Strategies for Stabilizing Mood and Enhancing Well, Being

Bipolar disorder is a complex mental health condition characterized by extreme mood swings, including manic highs and depressive lows. While there is no cure for bipolar disorder, effective management strategies can help individuals stabilize their mood, reduce the frequency and severity of episodes, and improve overall well, being. Managing bipolar disorder involves a combination of medication management, psychotherapy, lifestyle adjustments, and self, care practices tailored to the individual's unique needs.

Medication Management: Medications are often a cornerstone of bipolar disorder treatment. Mood stabilizers, such as lithium, valproate, or lamotrigine, help to prevent mood swings and stabilize mood. Antipsychotic medications may be prescribed during acute manic or mixed episodes. Antidepressants, cautiously used in combination with mood stabilizers, can help manage depressive symptoms. It is essential to work closely with a healthcare professional to find the most effective medication regimen and adjust dosages as needed. Adhering to the prescribed medication schedule and communicating any side effects or concerns to the healthcare provider are crucial for successful medication management.

Psychotherapy: Psychotherapy plays a critical role in managing bipolar disorder. Cognitive, behavioral therapy (CBT) focuses on identifying and modifying negative thought patterns and behaviors associated with mood episodes. It helps individuals develop coping strategies, manage stressors, and improve problem, solving skills. Family, focused therapy (FFT) involves working with the individual and their family members to enhance communication, reduce conflict, and improve support systems. Interpersonal and social rhythm therapy (IPSRT) emphasizes maintaining regular routines and managing social relationships to promote mood stability. Engaging in psychotherapy provides individuals with valuable tools to manage their symptoms, regulate emotions, and enhance resilience.

Lifestyle Adjustments: Making lifestyle adjustments is essential in managing bipolar disorder. Establishing regular sleep patterns, maintaining a balanced diet, and engaging in regular exercise are important components of a healthy lifestyle. Sleep hygiene practices, such as setting consistent bedtimes and avoiding stimulants close to bedtime, can promote better sleep quality. A nutritious diet rich in fruits, vegetables, whole grains, and lean proteins can provide the body with essential nutrients for optimal functioning. Regular physical activity, such as walking, jogging, or yoga, can help reduce stress, improve mood, and enhance overall well, being.

Stress Management: Stress can trigger mood episodes in individuals with bipolar disorder. Learning effective stress management techniques is crucial for preventing or minimizing the impact of stress on mood. Engaging in relaxation exercises, such as deep breathing, meditation, or mindfulness, can help reduce anxiety and promote relaxation. Participating in activities that bring joy and relaxation, such as hobbies, art, or spending time in nature, can serve as outlets for stress relief. Developing healthy coping mechanisms, such as seeking social support, practicing problem, solving, or engaging in therapy, can help individuals navigate stressful situations more effectively.

Social Support: Building a strong support network is invaluable in managing bipolar disorder. Seeking support from trusted family members, friends, or support groups can provide understanding, empathy, and encouragement. Support groups specifically tailored for individuals with bipolar disorder offer the opportunity to connect with others who share similar experiences, share coping strategies, and provide validation. Social support can help individuals feel less isolated, provide practical advice, and foster a sense of community.

Self, Care Practices: Engaging in self, care activities is essential for overall well, being. Self, care involves taking time to prioritize one's physical, emotional, and mental health. Engaging in activities that bring joy, relaxation, and fulfillment, such as reading, listening to music, practicing hobbies, or spending time in nature, can contribute to improved mood and well, being.

Developing a treatment plan

Developing a Treatment Plan for Bipolar Disorders: A Comprehensive Approach

Developing an effective treatment plan is crucial in managing bipolar disorders and promoting long, term stability and well, being. A comprehensive treatment plan takes into account the unique needs and preferences of individuals, considering the severity of symptoms, functional impairment, and treatment response. It typically includes a combination of medication management, psychotherapy, lifestyle adjustments, and support systems tailored to the specific challenges associated with bipolar disorders.

Assessment and Diagnosis: The treatment planning process begins with a thorough assessment and diagnosis of bipolar disorders. Mental health professionals conduct comprehensive evaluations, considering the individual's medical history, family history, and symptomatology. They gather information about the presence and severity of manic, hypomanic, and depressive episodes, as well as any associated functional impairment. Accurate assessment is essential in determining the appropriate treatment approach and establishing baseline measurements for tracking progress.

Medication Management: Medications, such as mood stabilizers, antipsychotics, and antidepressants, play a crucial role in stabilizing mood and managing symptoms. Working closely with a psychiatrist or other prescribing healthcare professional, individuals and their treatment team identify the most appropriate medication regimen based on the individual's symptom profile, medical history, and treatment response. Regular follow, up appointments allow for monitoring of medication effectiveness, adjustment of dosages if necessary, and management of any side effects. Medication management is a dynamic process that requires ongoing assessment and collaboration.

Psychotherapy: Psychotherapy is an integral component of bipolar disorder treatment. Various approaches, such as cognitive, behavioral therapy (CBT), family, focused therapy (FFT), and interpersonal and social rhythm therapy (IPSRT), are used to address different aspects of bipolar disorders. Individuals work with mental health professionals to develop coping strategies, manage stress, regulate emotions, and prevent relapse. The choice of psychotherapy approach is based on the individual's needs and treatment goals, with therapy sessions conducted on a regular basis to ensure consistent support and progress.

Lifestyle Adjustments: Making lifestyle adjustments is essential in managing bipolar disorders. Establishing a regular sleep schedule, maintaining a balanced diet, engaging in regular exercise, and avoiding substance abuse are critical factors in stabilizing mood and promoting overall well, being. Healthcare professionals provide guidance and support in adopting healthy lifestyle habits. Individuals are encouraged to develop routines that prioritize self, care, stress management, and a healthy work, life balance. Regular communication and feedback with the treatment team help identify potential areas for improvement and adjustment.

Social Support: Building a strong support system is vital in managing bipolar disorders. Friends, family members, and support groups provide understanding, empathy, and encouragement. Support groups specifically tailored for individuals with bipolar disorders offer a safe space for sharing experiences, learning coping strategies, and fostering a sense of community. Treatment plans often include recommendations for individuals to actively seek and engage in social support, both online and offline.

Regular Monitoring and Evaluation: Treatment plans should include mechanisms for regular monitoring and evaluation of progress. This involves tracking symptoms, functional impairment, and treatment response over time. Mental health professionals utilize standardized assessment tools, self, report measures, and clinical interviews to assess the effectiveness of interventions and make adjustments as necessary. Regular check, ins with the treatment team allow for ongoing communication, identification of any emerging concerns, and adjustment of treatment strategies as needed.

Crisis and Relapse Planning: Developing a crisis and relapse plan is essential to address potential setbacks or acute episodes. The plan outlines steps to take in the event of a crisis, including whom to contact, when to seek emergency services, and strategies for self, care and safety. Crisis plans may involve input from mental health professionals, family members, and individuals themselves.

Identifying and managing triggers

Identifying and Managing Triggers in Bipolar Disorders: Nurturing Stability and Well, Being

Bipolar disorders are characterized by extreme mood swings, including manic highs and depressive lows. While the exact causes of bipolar disorders are still being studied, it is widely recognized that certain triggers can contribute to the onset or exacerbation of mood episodes. Identifying and effectively managing these triggers is crucial for individuals with bipolar disorders to achieve and maintain stability. By recognizing and implementing strategies to mitigate the impact of triggers, individuals can better manage their condition and enhance overall well, being.

Understanding Triggers: Triggers are external or internal factors that can disrupt the delicate balance of mood in individuals with bipolar disorders. External triggers include stressful life events, major life changes, disruptions in routines, interpersonal conflicts, and substance abuse. Internal triggers encompass changes in sleep patterns, disruptions in circadian rhythms, hormonal fluctuations, and negative thought patterns. By recognizing and understanding the various triggers that can influence their mood, individuals are empowered to take proactive steps to manage and minimize their impact.

Self, Awareness and Monitoring: Self, awareness is a key component of identifying triggers. Individuals are encouraged to pay attention to their thoughts, emotions, physical sensations, and behaviors. Keeping a mood diary or utilizing mood, tracking apps can help individuals recognize patterns and identify potential triggers. By monitoring their moods and noting any changes or fluctuations, individuals can gain insights into the factors that contribute to mood shifts and episodes. This self, monitoring process can be instrumental in developing personalized strategies for managing triggers.

Stress Management: Stress is a significant trigger for mood episodes in bipolar disorders. Developing effective stress management techniques is crucial in minimizing its impact. Engaging in stress, reduction activities such as exercise, mindfulness meditation, deep breathing exercises, or engaging in hobbies can help individuals regulate their stress levels. Implementing time management strategies, setting realistic goals, and establishing boundaries can also reduce stress and create a more balanced lifestyle. Building a strong support network and seeking social support during stressful times can provide individuals with the necessary emotional support and guidance.

Sleep Hygiene: Sleep disturbances and disruptions in sleep patterns are commonly associated with mood episodes in bipolar disorders. Establishing a regular sleep schedule and practicing good sleep hygiene is essential in promoting stability. Individuals are encouraged to create a soothing bedtime routine, maintain a comfortable sleep environment, and avoid stimulating activities close to bedtime. Consistency in sleep, wake times, even on weekends or during vacations, can help regulate circadian rhythms and reduce the risk of triggering mood episodes. Seeking professional help for sleep difficulties, such as insomnia, can also contribute to better sleep quality.

Healthy Lifestyle Choices: Making healthy lifestyle choices is important in managing bipolar disorders and reducing the impact of triggers. Adopting a balanced diet rich in whole foods, maintaining regular exercise routines, and avoiding excessive alcohol or drug use contribute to overall well, being. Proper nutrition and regular physical activity support brain health and help regulate mood. Engaging in activities that promote relaxation, such as yoga, art, or spending time in nature, can also be beneficial in managing triggers and promoting a sense of calm.

Psychoeducation and Therapy: Psychoeducation is a crucial component of managing triggers in bipolar disorders. By educating themselves about their condition, individuals can gain a better understanding of the triggers that may affect them. Learning about the connection between sleep, stress, lifestyle, and mood episodes helps individuals develop strategies for managing and mitigating the impact of triggers. Engaging in therapy, such as cognitive, behavioral therapy (CBT) or interpersonal therapy, provides individuals with tools and coping mechanisms to effectively manage triggers and regulate their emotional responses.

Coping with symptoms: self

,

help strategies

Bipolar disorders are characterized by the presence of manic and depressive episodes, which can significantly impact an individual's daily life. While medications and therapy are essential components of treatment, individuals with bipolar disorders can also utilize self, help strategies to cope with their symptoms and enhance their overall well, being. By adopting effective self, care practices and implementing specific coping techniques, individuals can better manage their condition and lead fulfilling lives.

Establishing a Routine: Maintaining a structured routine is crucial in managing bipolar disorders. Establishing regular sleep patterns, meal times, and daily activities can help stabilize mood and prevent disruptions. Consistency in routines helps regulate the body's internal clock, promoting better sleep quality and stability. Creating a schedule that includes time for self, care, exercise, work, and leisure activities can provide a sense of structure and control over one's day.

Stress Reduction Techniques: Stress can trigger mood episodes in individuals with bipolar disorders. Developing effective stress reduction techniques is essential for managing symptoms. Engaging in activities such as deep breathing exercises, meditation, mindfulness, and progressive muscle relaxation can promote relaxation and reduce stress levels. Engaging in hobbies, listening to music, or spending time in nature are also effective ways to alleviate stress and improve overall well, being.

Building a Support Network: Building a strong support network is invaluable in coping with bipolar disorders. Surrounding oneself with understanding and supportive individuals can provide comfort and encouragement during difficult times. Family members, close friends, or support groups can offer a listening ear, practical advice, and a sense of belonging. Online communities and forums dedicated to bipolar disorders can also provide a platform for individuals to connect and share experiences.

Practicing Healthy Communication: Effective communication skills are crucial in managing relationships and minimizing conflicts, which can trigger mood episodes. Developing assertiveness skills and expressing emotions and needs in a clear and respectful manner can contribute to healthier interpersonal interactions. Learning active listening techniques and seeking to understand others' perspectives can enhance communication and foster positive relationships.

Monitoring Mood and Early Warning Signs: Regularly monitoring mood and identifying early warning signs of mood episodes can help individuals intervene and manage symptoms before they escalate. Keeping a mood journal or using mood tracking apps allows individuals to track their mood patterns over time and identify triggers. Recognizing early warning signs, such as changes in sleep patterns, increased irritability, or racing thoughts, can prompt individuals to implement self, care strategies or seek professional support.

Engaging in Regular Exercise: Regular physical exercise has been shown to have positive effects on mood and overall well, being. Engaging in activities such as walking, jogging, dancing, or yoga can help regulate stress hormones, improve sleep quality, and boost mood. Exercise releases endorphins, which are natural mood enhancers, and provides a healthy outlet for stress and tension.

Practicing Mindfulness and Self, Reflection: Mindfulness techniques, such as meditation or deep breathing exercises, can help individuals become more aware of their thoughts, emotions, and bodily sensations. By cultivating mindfulness, individuals can observe their experiences without judgment and develop a greater sense of self, awareness. Engaging in self, reflection allows individuals to identify patterns, triggers, and coping strategies that work best for them. It promotes self, understanding and empowers individuals to make positive changes in their lives.

Seeking Continued Education and Support: Educating oneself about bipolar disorders and staying informed about the latest research and treatment options is crucial. Continued education helps individuals become active participants in their treatment and empowers them to make informed decisions about their mental health. Seeking ongoing support from mental health professionals, attending therapy sessions, and actively participating in treatment planning contribute to better self, management and long, term stability.

Chapter Seven

The Role of Support Networks

The Role of Support Networks in Bipolar Disorders: Nurturing Understanding, Encouragement, and Resilience

Bipolar disorders can significantly impact an individual's life, making the presence of a strong support network invaluable. Support networks encompass family, friends, healthcare professionals, and support groups. These networks play a vital role in providing understanding, encouragement, and practical assistance to individuals living with bipolar disorders. The involvement of supportive individuals can enhance treatment outcomes, improve overall well, being, and foster resilience in the face of the challenges associated with bipolar disorders.

Emotional Support: Emotional support is crucial for individuals with bipolar disorders. Understanding family members and friends can provide a safe space for individuals to express their emotions, fears, and concerns. The availability of compassionate listeners can alleviate feelings of isolation and offer validation. Emotional support helps individuals feel heard and understood, reducing the stigma often associated with mental health conditions. Support networks can provide reassurance during difficult times and empower individuals to seek help when needed.

Practical Assistance: Practical assistance from support networks can be instrumental in managing daily life and reducing stress levels. Loved ones can assist with tasks such as managing finances, household chores, or transportation to medical appointments. Practical support allows individuals to focus on their well, being and treatment without the additional burden of overwhelming responsibilities. Support networks can also offer assistance in organizing treatment plans, scheduling appointments, and keeping track of medication regimens.

Education and Understanding: Support networks can contribute to education and understanding about bipolar disorders. By learning about the condition, loved ones can gain insights into the symptoms, triggers, and treatment approaches associated with bipolar disorders. Education helps dispel myths, reduce stigma, and fosters empathy and support. Understanding the challenges faced by individuals with bipolar disorders can enhance communication, foster healthy relationships, and promote a more supportive and inclusive environment.

Crisis Intervention: During periods of crisis, support networks play a critical role in providing immediate assistance. Loved ones can be vigilant for warning signs of a crisis, such as severe mood swings or suicidal ideation, and help individuals access appropriate care. Support networks can guide individuals to emergency services or accompany them to healthcare facilities. By having trusted individuals available to intervene during crises, individuals with bipolar disorders can receive timely and appropriate support.

Encouragement and Motivation: Encouragement and motivation from support networks are essential for individuals with bipolar disorders. Loved ones can provide positive reinforcement, acknowledge progress, and celebrate achievements, no matter how small. Encouragement helps individuals stay motivated in their treatment journey and fosters a sense of hope and resilience. Support networks can provide reminders of self, care practices, treatment adherence, and the importance of seeking professional help when needed.

Support Groups: Support groups dedicated to bipolar disorders offer individuals the opportunity to connect with others who share similar experiences. These groups provide a safe and non, judgmental space for individuals to share their thoughts, concerns, and coping strategies. Support groups can provide valuable insights, practical advice, and a sense of community. Individuals can learn from each other's experiences, gain perspective, and find comfort in knowing that they are not alone in their journey.

Collaboration with Healthcare Professionals: Support networks collaborate with healthcare professionals to ensure coordinated care for individuals with bipolar disorders. Loved ones can accompany individuals to medical appointments, help communicate concerns, and actively participate in the treatment planning process. Collaboration between support networks and healthcare professionals fosters a comprehensive approach to treatment, considering the perspectives and needs of both the individual and their support system.

Promoting Self, Advocacy: Support networks play a vital role in empowering individuals with bipolar disorders to become self, advocates. Loved ones can encourage individuals to voice their needs, ask questions, and actively participate in treatment decisions.

Family and friends: providing support and understanding

Family and Friends: Providing Support and Understanding for Individuals with Bipolar Disorders

Family and friends play a crucial role in the lives of individuals with bipolar disorders. Their support and understanding can make a significant difference in the well, being and recovery of their loved ones. By providing a nurturing environment, educating themselves about the condition, and offering empathy and assistance, family and friends can create a strong support system that promotes stability and resilience in individuals living with bipolar disorders.

Creating a Nurturing Environment: Creating a nurturing environment is fundamental to supporting individuals with bipolar disorders. Loved ones can foster a safe and understanding atmosphere that encourages open communication and self, expression. Acceptance and non, judgmental attitudes create an environment where individuals feel comfortable discussing their experiences and seeking help when needed. A nurturing environment reduces stigma, encourages treatment adherence, and promotes overall well, being.

Educating Themselves about Bipolar Disorders: Educating themselves about bipolar disorders is a critical step for family and friends. Learning about the symptoms, triggers, and treatment options associated with bipolar disorders can help loved ones understand the experiences of their family member or friend. Education promotes empathy, reduces misconceptions, and enables more informed support. By staying up, to, date with research and seeking information from reputable sources, family and friends can better comprehend the challenges faced by individuals with bipolar disorders.

Active Listening and Empathy: Active listening and empathy are essential skills for family and friends supporting individuals with bipolar disorders. Listening attentively, without interruption or judgment, conveys a sense of understanding and validation. Showing empathy by acknowledging the emotions and experiences of their loved ones helps individuals feel heard and supported. Empathetic responses, such as "I can understand why you feel that way" or "I'm here for you," foster a deeper connection and create a safe space for open dialogue.

Providing Practical Assistance: Practical assistance from family and friends can alleviate some of the challenges faced by individuals with bipolar disorders. Offering help with daily tasks, such as household chores, childcare, or errands, lightens the burden and allows individuals to focus on their well, being. Assisting with medication management, appointment scheduling, or attending medical appointments together can also provide practical support. Small gestures of assistance can make a significant difference in reducing stress and promoting stability.

Encouraging Treatment Adherence: Encouraging treatment adherence is a vital role for family and friends. Loved ones can remind individuals to take their medications regularly, attend therapy sessions, and follow through with recommended self, care practices. Reinforcing the importance of treatment and acknowledging the efforts made by their loved ones fosters motivation and commitment to recovery. Family and friends can actively participate in treatment discussions, ask questions, and support treatment decisions.

Recognizing Early Warning Signs: Family and friends who are closely involved with individuals with bipolar disorders can help identify early warning signs of mood episodes. By recognizing subtle changes in behavior, sleep patterns, or mood, loved ones can intervene early and assist in implementing coping strategies. Communication and collaboration with healthcare professionals are crucial in developing a plan to manage potential mood shifts effectively.

Managing Communication and Conflict: Effective communication and conflict management skills are essential in supporting individuals with bipolar disorders. Loved ones can learn strategies for constructive communication, such as using "I" statements, active listening, and avoiding blame or criticism. Open and honest conversations allow for the expression of concerns, fears, and needs. Conflict resolution techniques, such as finding compromises or seeking professional mediation, can help minimize stress and maintain healthy relationships.

Practicing Self, Care: Supporting individuals with bipolar disorders also requires self, care for family and friends. Caring for oneself ensures that they have the emotional and physical resources to provide support effectively.

Support groups and peer networks

Support Groups and Peer Networks: Strengthening Connections and Empowering Individuals with Bipolar Disorders

Support groups and peer networks play a vital role in the lives of individuals with bipolar disorders. These communities provide a safe and understanding space where individuals can connect with others who share similar experiences. By fostering a sense of belonging, offering practical advice, and promoting emotional support, support groups and peer networks contribute to the overall well, being and resilience of individuals living with bipolar disorders.

Creating a Safe and Understanding Space: Support groups and peer networks create a safe and understanding environment for individuals with bipolar disorders. Within these communities, individuals can freely express their thoughts, emotions, and concerns without fear of judgment or stigma. Sharing experiences, challenges, and successes with others who can relate helps individuals feel validated and less alone in their journey. The acceptance and empathy found in support groups and peer networks create a foundation for healing and growth.

Sharing Knowledge and Information: Support groups and peer networks serve as valuable sources of knowledge and information. Participants can exchange practical advice, strategies for coping with symptoms, and insights into treatment options. Sharing personal experiences and lessons learned can provide individuals with valuable perspectives and new approaches to managing their condition. Peer, led discussions and educational sessions contribute to a collaborative learning environment that empowers individuals to make informed decisions about their treatment and well, being.

Emotional Support and Empathy: Emotional support and empathy are at the core of support groups and peer networks. Being surrounded by individuals who truly understand the challenges and emotions associated with bipolar disorders can offer immense comfort and encouragement. Participants can provide empathetic listening, validation, and encouragement, which can alleviate feelings of isolation and foster hope. By sharing in each other's journeys, individuals gain a sense of community and the reassurance that they are not alone in their experiences.

Practical Coping Strategies: Support groups and peer networks offer opportunities for individuals to learn and develop practical coping strategies. Participants can share techniques for managing mood swings, stress, and everyday challenges. Strategies such as mindfulness exercises, relaxation techniques, and effective communication skills can be taught and practiced within the group. The collective wisdom of the community provides individuals with a wide range of tools and resources to navigate the ups and downs of bipolar disorders.

Learning from Role Models: Within support groups and peer networks, individuals can find role models who have successfully managed their bipolar disorders. These individuals serve as sources of inspiration, offering hope and demonstrating that a fulfilling life is possible despite the challenges. Witnessing the resilience and achievements of others can instill confidence and motivation in individuals who may be struggling. Role models provide tangible evidence that recovery and stability are attainable goals.

Enhancing Self, Esteem and Self, Advocacy: Support groups and peer networks empower individuals to develop a strong sense of self, esteem and self, advocacy. By sharing their stories and receiving validation from others, participants can gain a better understanding of their strengths and resilience. They can also build assertiveness skills, learn to articulate their needs, and advocate for themselves within their treatment and personal lives. Support groups and peer networks provide individuals with the confidence and skills necessary to actively participate in their own well, being.

Promoting Accountability and Responsibility: Support groups and peer networks foster a sense of accountability and responsibility among participants. By openly discussing their goals, treatment plans, and progress, individuals are encouraged to take ownership of their journey towards stability. The shared commitment to self, improvement creates a culture of accountability, where individuals inspire and motivate each other to adhere to their treatment regimens, engage in self, care practices, and make healthy lifestyle choices.

Long, Term Relationships and Social Connections: Support groups and peer networks often lead to the formation of long, term relationships and social connections.

Online resources and communities

Online Resources and Communities: Expanding Support and Knowledge for Individuals with Bipolar Disorders

In the digital age, online resources and communities have become valuable platforms for individuals with bipolar disorders to connect, seek support, and access information. These online spaces offer a wealth of resources, educational materials, and platforms for communication, creating a virtual support network that transcends geographical boundaries. Through online resources and communities, individuals with bipolar disorders can enhance their understanding of the condition, find solace in shared experiences, and access a supportive community that empowers their journey towards stability and well, being.

Access to Information: Online resources provide a wealth of information about bipolar disorders. Websites, blogs, and reputable online sources offer comprehensive and up, to, date information about symptoms, treatment options, coping strategies, and research developments. Individuals can educate themselves about the condition, its underlying causes, and the various approaches to managing bipolar disorders. Online resources also provide guidance on finding healthcare professionals, treatment centers, and local support groups. Accessible information equips individuals with the knowledge necessary to make informed decisions about their treatment and self, care.

Online Support Groups: Online support groups specifically tailored to bipolar disorders create a supportive community for individuals to share their experiences, concerns, and insights. These groups foster a sense of belonging, as individuals can connect with others who understand the unique challenges of living with bipolar disorders. Through message boards, forums, and social media platforms, individuals can seek advice, ask questions, and offer support to one another. Online support groups provide a safe space for open discussions, enabling individuals to express themselves without fear of judgment or stigma.

Peer Mentorship: Online communities often feature peer mentorship programs, where individuals with lived experience of bipolar disorders offer guidance, encouragement, and practical advice to those who are newly diagnosed or struggling with their condition. Peer mentors can provide valuable insights into managing symptoms, navigating treatment options, and finding resources. Peer mentorship fosters a sense of hope and resilience, as individuals can witness the successes and achievements of those who have successfully managed their bipolar disorders.

Online Therapy and Counseling: Online therapy platforms and virtual counseling services have emerged as convenient options for individuals with bipolar disorders seeking professional support. Through secure video conferencing or messaging systems, individuals can connect with licensed therapists or counselors who specialize in bipolar disorders. Online therapy offers flexibility, accessibility, and confidentiality, making it a viable option for those who may face challenges accessing in, person therapy. These platforms provide individualized treatment plans, evidence, based interventions, and ongoing support from qualified mental health professionals.

Education and Awareness Campaigns: Online platforms play a crucial role in raising awareness about bipolar disorders and promoting mental health education. Organizations and advocacy groups use websites, social media, and online campaigns to disseminate accurate information, challenge stigma, and promote understanding. Online platforms serve as powerful tools for sharing personal stories, organizing virtual events, and promoting mental health initiatives. By increasing awareness and understanding, online communities contribute to reducing the stigma associated with bipolar disorders.

Online Self, Help Resources: Online self, help resources, such as guided self, help modules, interactive tools, and mobile applications, offer individuals with bipolar disorders practical strategies for managing their symptoms. These resources often provide psychoeducation, cognitive, behavioral techniques, and self, assessment tools to enhance self, awareness and self, management. Online self, help resources can assist individuals in developing coping skills, managing stress, regulating sleep patterns, and monitoring mood fluctuations. These interactive platforms empower individuals to take an active role in their own well, being.

Online Education and Webinars: Online education platforms and webinars offer individuals with bipolar disorders the opportunity to participate in educational programs from the comfort of their own homes.

Chapter Eight

Bipolar Disorder and Relationships

Bipolar Disorder and Relationships: Navigating the Challenges and Fostering Understanding

Bipolar disorder can significantly impact not only the individuals diagnosed but also their relationships with loved ones. The unpredictable mood swings, intense emotions, and varying energy levels associated with bipolar disorder can pose unique challenges for maintaining healthy and fulfilling relationships. However, with understanding, communication, and support, individuals with bipolar disorder and their partners, family members, and friends can navigate these challenges and build strong, resilient relationships that promote overall well, being.

Educating Loved Ones: Education is key to fostering understanding and empathy within relationships affected by bipolar disorder. Loved ones should take the initiative to learn about the condition, including its symptoms, triggers, and treatment options. By educating themselves, they can gain insights into the experiences and challenges faced by individuals with bipolar disorder. Understanding that mood swings are a result of a medical condition, rather than a personal attack, helps loved ones respond with compassion and support.

Open and Honest Communication: Communication is essential in any relationship, but it becomes even more critical when one person is living with bipolar disorder. Open and honest communication allows individuals to express their feelings, concerns, and needs in a safe and non, judgmental environment. Both individuals should actively listen to each other, seeking to understand rather than criticize. Developing effective communication skills, such as using "I" statements and avoiding blame, creates a foundation for healthy dialogue and problem, solving.

Establishing Boundaries and Routines: Establishing clear boundaries and routines can provide stability and predictability within the relationship. Individuals with bipolar disorder may benefit from maintaining a structured daily routine that includes consistent sleep patterns, meal times, and medication schedules. Partners and loved ones can support this by creating an environment that encourages adherence to these routines. Setting healthy boundaries, such as recognizing when personal space is needed or establishing guidelines for conflict resolution, helps maintain balance and respect within the relationship.

Supporting Treatment and Self, Care: Loved ones can play a crucial role in supporting the individual's treatment and self, care efforts. Encouraging adherence to medication regimens, attending therapy sessions together, and actively participating in treatment discussions demonstrates commitment and support. Partners and loved ones can also assist in recognizing early warning signs of mood episodes and helping individuals implement self, care strategies. By showing a genuine interest in the individual's well, being, loved ones contribute to the overall management of bipolar disorder.

Coping Strategies for Loved Ones: Caring for someone with bipolar disorder can be emotionally challenging, and loved ones need to prioritize their own well, being as well. Developing personal coping strategies, such as seeking support from friends or joining caregiver support groups, is essential. These strategies provide an outlet to express concerns, share experiences, and gain insights from others who are in similar situations.

Taking time for self, care, engaging in activities that bring joy and relaxation, and setting realistic expectations can help loved ones maintain their own mental and emotional health.

Seeking Couples Therapy: Couples therapy can provide a safe and supportive environment for individuals with bipolar disorder and their partners to address relationship challenges. A therapist experienced in working with bipolar disorder can help couples improve communication, manage conflicts, and develop strategies for navigating mood episodes. Couples therapy also provides a space for both individuals to express their concerns, fears, and goals, fostering a deeper understanding of each other's experiences.

Developing a Support Network: Building a support network beyond the romantic relationship is crucial for both individuals. Loved ones can help create and nurture a support system that includes friends, family members, and support groups. Encouraging the individual with bipolar disorder to connect with others who share similar experiences can provide a sense of belonging and validation.

Communication and conflict resolution

Communication and Conflict Resolution: Nurturing Healthy Relationships in the Context of Bipolar Disorders

Effective communication and conflict resolution skills are vital for maintaining healthy relationships, particularly when one or both individuals are living with bipolar disorder. The unique challenges posed by the condition, such as mood swings and intense emotions, require a compassionate and understanding approach to communication. By developing open lines of communication, actively listening, and implementing effective conflict resolution strategies, individuals and their loved ones can foster understanding, strengthen their relationships, and navigate challenges in a supportive and constructive manner.

Establishing Open Lines of Communication: Open communication is the foundation of a healthy relationship. This is especially important when one person has bipolar disorder. Encourage regular and honest conversations about feelings, concerns, and needs. Creating a safe and non, judgmental space allows individuals to express themselves without fear of rejection or criticism. Both partners should strive to be active listeners, fully present and attentive to what the other person is saying. Effective communication builds trust and strengthens the connection between individuals.

Using "I" Statements: When discussing sensitive topics or expressing emotions, using "I" statements can promote understanding and minimize defensiveness. "I" statements allow individuals to take ownership of their feelings and experiences, reducing the likelihood of blame or accusation. For example, instead of saying, "You always make me angry," one could say, "I feel upset when certain things happen." This approach fosters empathy and encourages the listener to reflect on their behavior rather than becoming defensive.

Active Listening and Empathy: Active listening is an essential skill in effective communication. It involves giving the speaker undivided attention, maintaining eye contact, and acknowledging their feelings and perspective. Avoid interrupting or jumping to s. Reflective listening, paraphrasing, and asking clarifying questions can demonstrate genuine interest and understanding. Cultivating empathy allows individuals to truly connect with their partner's experiences, fostering compassion and emotional support.

Timing and Environment: Consider the timing and environment when engaging in important conversations or addressing conflicts. Choose a time when both individuals are calm and receptive. Avoid initiating discussions during moments of high stress or when one person is experiencing a mood episode. Create a comfortable and private space where both individuals feel safe to express themselves openly. Minimizing distractions, such as turning off electronic devices, helps ensure full engagement in the conversation.

Active Problem, Solving: Conflict is a natural part of any relationship, but it can be more challenging when bipolar disorder is involved. Engaging in active problem, solving techniques allows individuals to work together to find mutually beneficial solutions. Focus on the specific issue at hand and brainstorm potential solutions. Encourage creativity and flexibility in exploring different perspectives. Compromise and negotiation are key components of effective conflict resolution, aiming for resolutions that respect both individuals' needs and boundaries.

Seeking Professional Support: In some cases, couples may benefit from seeking professional support in navigating communication challenges and conflict resolution. Couples therapy provides a neutral and structured environment where a trained therapist can facilitate effective communication and offer guidance on managing conflicts. Therapists experienced in working with bipolar disorder can provide insight into the unique dynamics within the relationship and offer strategies tailored to the specific circumstances.

Practice Emotional Regulation Techniques: Emotional regulation is vital in managing conflicts effectively. Individuals with bipolar disorder can employ specific techniques, such as deep breathing exercises, mindfulness, or engaging in physical activities, to manage heightened emotions. Taking a short break or engaging in self, soothing activities can also provide the space needed to calm down before addressing conflicts. Encouraging these techniques as part of a joint effort can help individuals manage intense emotions and improve communication during challenging moments.

Maintaining healthy boundaries

Maintaining Healthy Boundaries: Nurturing Relationships in the Context of Bipolar Disorders

Establishing and maintaining healthy boundaries is crucial for individuals with bipolar disorder and their loved ones. Bipolar disorder can affect emotions, energy levels, and behavior, making it essential to define and respect personal limits within relationships. By fostering self, care, promoting autonomy, and effectively communicating boundaries, individuals can cultivate relationships that are supportive, respectful, and conducive to overall well, being.

Understanding Personal Needs: Recognizing and understanding personal needs is the first step in establishing healthy boundaries. Individuals with bipolar disorder should assess their emotional, physical, and mental well, being regularly. Identifying triggers, stressors, and limitations can help define boundaries that protect their overall stability. Taking time for self, reflection and self, awareness allows individuals to recognize when they need space, support, or assistance.

Communicating Boundaries: Open communication is essential in defining and maintaining boundaries. Individuals should express their needs, limits, and expectations clearly and assertively to their loved ones. It is important to communicate boundaries in a non, confrontational manner, emphasizing the intention to maintain a healthy and balanced relationship. Encourage an open dialogue, inviting loved ones to share their perspectives and concerns as well.

Respecting Personal Space: Respecting personal space is crucial for individuals with bipolar disorder. This includes physical, emotional, and psychological boundaries. Allowing individuals to have time alone or engage in activities they enjoy without feeling guilty or pressured is essential for self, care. Loved ones should understand and support these needs, recognizing that personal space is vital for maintaining stability and well, being.

Differentiating between the Person and the Illness: It is important to differentiate between the individual and their bipolar disorder. Loved ones should recognize that mood swings, intense emotions, or behavioral changes associated with bipolar disorder do not define the person's character or intentions. By separating the person from their illness, loved ones can avoid taking mood fluctuations personally and maintain healthy boundaries in their interactions.

Establishing Emotional Boundaries: Emotional boundaries are crucial for individuals with bipolar disorder to protect their emotional well, being. Loved ones should be mindful of their own emotions and not rely solely on the individual with bipolar disorder for emotional support. Encourage individuals to seek professional help or engage in support networks to share their experiences and emotions. Establishing emotional boundaries ensures that the responsibility for emotional support is shared and prevents emotional burnout.

Setting Limits on Responsibilities: Individuals with bipolar disorder may require additional support at times, but it is important to set realistic limits on the level of responsibility assumed by loved ones. Loved ones should avoid assuming the role of the primary caregiver or becoming overly involved in managing the individual's condition. Encourage independence and self, management while being available as a support system.

Recognizing Warning Signs: Loved ones should familiarize themselves with the warning signs of mood episodes and respect the individual's boundaries during these times. It is crucial to give the person space when needed and avoid triggering situations or discussions. Recognizing warning signs allows loved ones to respond appropriately and supportively while maintaining appropriate boundaries.

Seeking Support Networks: Encourage individuals with bipolar disorder and their loved ones to seek support from external networks. Joining support groups or engaging in therapy can provide additional guidance and understanding from individuals who have similar experiences. Support networks offer a safe space for sharing challenges, coping strategies, and mutual support, reinforcing the importance of boundaries and self, care.

Continuous Evaluation and Adjustment: Boundaries should be continuously evaluated and adjusted as needed. As individuals grow and change, their boundaries may evolve. Regular communication and reassessment of boundaries within relationships help ensure that they remain effective and supportive. This ongoing process allows individuals to adapt to the challenges posed by bipolar disorder and maintain healthy and respectful interactions.

Intimacy, sexuality, and bipolar disorder

Intimacy, Sexuality, and Bipolar Disorder: Nurturing Healthy Relationships and Exploring Challenges

Intimacy and sexuality are important aspects of human relationships, but they can be uniquely impacted by bipolar disorder. The fluctuating moods, energy levels, and medication effects associated with bipolar disorder can pose challenges in maintaining a fulfilling and satisfying intimate life. However, with understanding, communication, and adaptation, individuals with bipolar disorder and their partners can navigate these challenges and nurture healthy, intimate relationships.

Understanding the Impact of Bipolar Disorder: It is crucial for individuals and their partners to understand how bipolar disorder can affect intimacy and sexuality. The condition's manic and depressive episodes, along with medication side effects, may lead to changes in libido, sexual desire, and energy levels. Recognizing that these fluctuations are part of the condition rather than a personal rejection can help reduce frustration and promote understanding.

Open and Honest Communication: Communication is key in any relationship, and it is especially important when discussing intimacy and sexuality in the context of bipolar disorder. Both individuals should feel comfortable expressing their needs, concerns, and desires openly and without judgment. Create a safe space where discussions can take place, allowing both partners to express their feelings and work together to find solutions that accommodate the challenges posed by bipolar disorder.

Timing and Energy Management: Bipolar disorder can impact energy levels and interfere with the ability to engage in sexual activities. Partners should be mindful of each other's energy levels and consider finding the right timing for intimacy. Planning activities during periods of increased energy or stability can help optimize experiences. It is important to respect each other's boundaries and not feel pressured to engage in sexual activities when one partner is not feeling up to it.

Exploring Non, Sexual Intimacy: Intimacy is not solely limited to sexual activities. Partners can focus on building emotional intimacy through non, sexual activities such as cuddling, holding hands, or engaging in deep conversations. These acts of affection can strengthen the emotional connection between partners and foster a sense of closeness and intimacy, even during periods when sexual activity may not be possible or desired.

Adjusting Expectations: It is important to adjust expectations regarding sexual frequency and performance. Bipolar disorder can result in unpredictable changes in libido and sexual function. Both partners should be willing to adapt to these changes and find alternative ways to maintain a satisfying intimate life. Openly discussing expectations, desires, and limitations can help set realistic goals and alleviate pressure or frustration.

Medication Effects and Sexual Side Effects: Medications used to manage bipolar disorder can sometimes have sexual side effects such as decreased libido, erectile dysfunction, or difficulties with orgasm. Individuals should discuss these potential side effects with their healthcare provider and explore alternative medications or dosage adjustments if necessary. Open communication with medical professionals can help address these issues and find solutions that minimize the impact on intimacy and sexual satisfaction.

Self, Care and Stress Management: Managing bipolar disorder requires individuals to prioritize self, care and stress management. Engaging in activities that promote overall well, being, such as regular exercise, quality sleep, and stress reduction techniques, can positively impact intimacy and sexual health. Encouraging each other to practice self, care and managing stress together as a team can foster a supportive environment that enhances the intimate relationship.

Seeking Professional Help: If intimacy and sexual difficulties persist and become a significant source of distress, individuals and their partners may consider seeking professional help. Sex therapists or couples counselors experienced in working with individuals with bipolar disorder can provide guidance, education, and techniques to address specific challenges. These professionals can offer tools and strategies to improve communication, rebuild intimacy, and navigate the impact of bipolar disorder on the intimate relationship.

Emotional Support and Understanding: Bipolar disorder can sometimes lead to emotional challenges that impact intimacy and sexuality.

Chapter Nine

Bipolar Disorder in Children and Adolescents

Bipolar Disorder in Children and Adolescents: Recognizing, Understanding, and Supporting Young Individuals

Bipolar disorder, typically associated with adults, can also manifest in children and adolescents. While the diagnosis of bipolar disorder in young individuals presents unique challenges, it is essential to recognize the signs, understand the impact, and provide appropriate support. By raising awareness, promoting early intervention, and fostering a comprehensive treatment approach, we can empower children and adolescents with bipolar disorder to manage their condition and lead fulfilling lives.

Recognizing the Signs: Bipolar disorder in children and adolescents can present differently from adults. Common symptoms include extreme mood swings, irritability, impulsive behavior, and difficulty regulating emotions. Children may experience intense episodes of euphoria (mania) or prolonged periods of sadness and hopelessness (depression). Sleep disturbances, changes in appetite, and problems with concentration and school performance are also possible indicators. Recognizing these signs early allows for timely intervention and support.

Challenges in Diagnosis: Diagnosing bipolar disorder in children and adolescents can be challenging due to overlapping symptoms with other mental health conditions and typical developmental changes. Additionally, young individuals may have difficulty articulating their experiences accurately. It requires a thorough evaluation by mental health professionals, including a comprehensive assessment of symptoms, family history, and functional impairment. Collaborating with parents, teachers, and caregivers is crucial to gather a comprehensive picture of the child's behavior and emotions.

The Impact of Bipolar Disorder on Development: Bipolar disorder can significantly impact a child or adolescent's overall development. It may affect academic performance, social interactions, and emotional well, being. The intense mood swings and impulsive behaviors can strain relationships with peers, family members, and educators. Young individuals with bipolar disorder may face challenges in maintaining stable friendships, participating in extracurricular activities, and achieving academic success. Early identification and intervention are vital to support healthy development.

Multidimensional Treatment Approach: The treatment of bipolar disorder in children and adolescents requires a multidimensional approach involving various professionals, including psychiatrists, therapists, and educators. Medication may be prescribed to stabilize mood fluctuations and manage symptoms. Psychosocial interventions, such as cognitive, behavioral therapy (CBT) and family therapy, play a crucial role in teaching coping skills, emotion regulation, and communication strategies. Collaborating with schools to provide academic accommodations and support is essential to address educational challenges.

Family Support and Education: A strong support system is crucial for children and adolescents with bipolar disorder. Educating family members about the condition, its symptoms, and treatment options helps them understand and provide appropriate support. Families can learn strategies to manage challenging behaviors, recognize warning signs, and create a supportive environment. Open communication, empathy, and fostering a non, judgmental atmosphere contribute to the emotional well, being of the young individual.

Psychoeducation for the Young Individual: Providing psychoeducation directly to the child or adolescent about their bipolar disorder can empower them to understand their condition and actively participate in their treatment. Age, appropriate explanations of the disorder, its impact on emotions and behaviors, and coping strategies can help young individuals develop a sense of self, awareness and self, advocacy. By involving them in the decision, making process and encouraging open discussions, they can develop resilience and become active participants in their treatment journey.

School, Based Support: Collaboration with schools is essential in addressing the educational needs of children and adolescents with bipolar disorder. Developing an individualized education plan (IEP) or a 504 plan that outlines academic accommodations and support services can ensure their educational needs are met. Regular communication between parents, mental health professionals, and educators helps monitor progress, identify challenges, and make necessary adjustments to support the student's well, being.

Early signs and diagnosis

Early Signs and Diagnosis: Identifying Bipolar Disorder in its Initial Stages

Bipolar disorder is a complex mental health condition characterized by extreme mood swings, ranging from manic highs to depressive lows. While bipolar disorder typically manifests in late adolescence or early adulthood, it is crucial to recognize the early signs and symptoms that may emerge before a formal diagnosis is made. Identifying bipolar disorder in its initial stages allows for timely intervention, appropriate treatment, and improved long, term outcomes. By understanding the early signs and seeking professional help, individuals can receive the support they need to manage their condition effectively.

Mood Instability: One of the primary indicators of bipolar disorder is noticeable fluctuations in mood. In the early stages, individuals may experience episodes of unexplained happiness, increased energy, and extreme enthusiasm. These episodes, known as hypomania, are milder forms of mania and can be mistaken for high spirits or a particularly joyful phase. Conversely, individuals may also exhibit periods of prolonged sadness, feelings of hopelessness, and a loss of interest in activities they once enjoyed, indicating early signs of depression.

Changes in Energy Levels and Sleep Patterns: Early signs of bipolar disorder may include alterations in energy levels and sleep patterns. During hypomanic or manic episodes, individuals may experience a surge in energy, requiring less sleep than usual. They may feel restless, engage in excessive activities, and experience a decreased need for restorative sleep. On the other hand, during depressive episodes, individuals may feel fatigued, lack energy, and experience disrupted sleep patterns, such as insomnia or excessive sleeping.

Impulsivity and Risk, Taking Behavior: Another early sign of bipolar disorder is an increase in impulsive behavior and risk, taking tendencies. Individuals may engage in excessive spending, participate in reckless activities, or make impulsive decisions without considering the consequences. These behaviors may be driven by the elevated mood and reduced inhibitions associated with hypomania or mania.

Changes in Concentration and Cognitive Functioning: Early signs of bipolar disorder may also be reflected in changes in cognitive functioning. During hypomanic or manic episodes, individuals may experience a heightened ability to concentrate, increased creativity, and a rapid flow of ideas. However, these periods may be accompanied by distractibility, racing thoughts, and difficulty focusing on tasks. Conversely, during depressive episodes, individuals may struggle with concentration, memory, and decision, making abilities.

Altered Social Interactions and Relationships: Bipolar disorder can impact social interactions and relationships, even in its early stages. Individuals may exhibit changes in behavior, such as increased talkativeness, rapid speech, and a heightened sense of self, importance during hypomanic or manic episodes. These changes may strain relationships and cause interpersonal conflicts. Additionally, during depressive episodes, individuals may withdraw from social activities, isolate themselves, and experience difficulty in maintaining healthy relationships.

Family History and Genetic Factors: Family history and genetic factors play a significant role in the development of bipolar disorder. If there is a family history of bipolar disorder or other mood disorders, individuals may be at a higher risk of developing the condition themselves. Awareness of the presence of bipolar disorder in the family can help identify potential early signs and prompt individuals to seek professional evaluation.

Seeking Professional Evaluation: Recognizing the early signs of bipolar disorder is crucial, but it is equally important to seek professional evaluation for an accurate diagnosis. Mental health professionals, such as psychiatrists or psychologists, are trained to assess symptoms, conduct comprehensive evaluations, and make an informed diagnosis. Seeking professional help ensures that individuals receive the appropriate treatment and support they need to manage their condition effectively.

Treatment options for young people

Treatment Options for Young People: Nurturing Well, being in the Management of Bipolar Disorder

Bipolar disorder, a complex mental health condition, can significantly impact the lives of young people. Timely and appropriate treatment is crucial in managing the symptoms and promoting well, being in this population. By adopting a comprehensive approach that encompasses medication, psychotherapy, and lifestyle modifications, young individuals with bipolar disorder can achieve stability, emotional resilience, and an improved quality of life.

Medication: Medication plays a vital role in managing bipolar disorder in young people. Mood stabilizers, such as lithium or anticonvulsants, are commonly prescribed to help regulate mood swings and prevent relapses. Medications may also include atypical antipsychotics or antidepressants, depending on the specific symptoms and severity of the condition. Close monitoring by a qualified healthcare professional is essential to ensure the effectiveness of the medication and minimize potential side effects.

Psychotherapy: Psychotherapy, or talk therapy, is an integral part of treatment for young individuals with bipolar disorder. Different types of therapy, such as cognitive, behavioral therapy (CBT), dialectical behavior therapy (DBT), and family, focused therapy (FFT), can provide valuable support and teach essential coping skills. CBT helps individuals identify and modify negative thought patterns and behaviors, while DBT focuses on emotion regulation and interpersonal effectiveness. FFT involves the family in therapy sessions to enhance communication, problem, solving, and overall family support.

Individual Therapy: Individual therapy offers young individuals a safe and confidential space to explore their thoughts, emotions, and experiences related to bipolar disorder. Therapists can help young people develop coping

strategies, improve self, esteem, and navigate the challenges associated with their condition. Additionally, therapists can assist in identifying triggers and warning signs of mood episodes, enabling individuals to take proactive measures to manage their symptoms effectively.

Family Involvement: The involvement of family members in the treatment process is essential for young individuals with bipolar disorder. Family therapy sessions can enhance communication, foster understanding, and provide a supportive environment. It allows family members to learn about the condition, recognize early signs of mood episodes, and develop strategies to support their loved one. Educating families about bipolar disorder and involving them in treatment decisions helps create a united front in managing the condition.

Peer Support: Peer support groups and programs specifically designed for young people with bipolar disorder can provide a sense of belonging, empathy, and understanding. Connecting with peers who share similar experiences can reduce feelings of isolation and provide valuable insights into managing the condition. Peer support groups offer a platform for sharing coping strategies, discussing challenges, and receiving validation and encouragement from others who can relate to their struggles.

School, Based Support: Collaborating with school professionals, such as teachers, counselors, and administrators, can help create a supportive educational environment for young individuals with bipolar disorder. Developing an individualized education plan (IEP) or a 504 plan ensures that the student receives appropriate academic accommodations and support. Regular communication with school staff allows for monitoring academic progress, addressing challenges, and implementing strategies to promote success in the educational setting.

Lifestyle Modifications: In addition to medical and therapeutic interventions, lifestyle modifications can significantly impact the well, being of young individuals with bipolar disorder. Maintaining a regular sleep schedule is crucial, as disrupted sleep patterns can exacerbate mood swings. Engaging in regular physical exercise can help manage stress, improve mood, and promote overall well, being. A balanced diet, avoidance of substance abuse, and healthy stress management techniques are important components of a healthy lifestyle for young individuals with bipolar disorder.

Relapse Prevention Planning: Developing a relapse prevention plan is important to empower young individuals with the skills to identify early warning signs and take proactive measures to prevent or minimize the impact of mood episodes.

Parenting strategies and family support

Parenting Strategies and Family Support: Nurturing Resilience in Children and Adolescents with Bipolar Disorder

Parenting a child or adolescent with bipolar disorder can present unique challenges for families. However, with the right strategies and support, parents can provide a nurturing and stable environment that promotes the well, being of their child. By implementing effective parenting techniques, seeking professional guidance, and fostering a supportive family environment, parents can help their child manage bipolar disorder and thrive.

Education and Understanding: Educating yourself about bipolar disorder is crucial in effectively parenting a child with the condition. Learn about the symptoms, triggers, and treatment options to better understand your child's experiences. Knowledge empowers you to provide appropriate support, recognize warning signs, and advocate for your child's needs.

Open Communication: Establishing open lines of communication with your child is vital. Encourage them to express their feelings, concerns, and experiences related to bipolar disorder. Listen attentively, validate their emotions, and avoid judgment. Creating a safe and supportive environment allows your child to feel heard, understood, and comfortable seeking help when needed.

Consistency and Structure: Children with bipolar disorder often benefit from a structured and predictable routine. Establish consistent mealtimes, bedtime routines, and daily schedules to provide stability and reduce anxiety. Clear expectations and consistent consequences for behavior help your child understand boundaries and foster a sense of security.

Emphasize Self, Care: Teach your child the importance of self, care to manage their condition effectively. Encourage activities that promote physical health, such as regular exercise, sufficient sleep, and a balanced diet. Promote healthy coping strategies like journaling, practicing mindfulness, or engaging in creative outlets. By modeling self, care and emphasizing its value, you encourage your child to prioritize their well, being.

Collaborate with Mental Health Professionals: Work collaboratively with mental health professionals who specialize in treating children and adolescents with bipolar disorder. Seek their guidance in developing an individualized treatment plan and addressing specific challenges your child may face. Regular check, ins with therapists, psychiatrists, or counselors ensure that your child's treatment remains comprehensive and tailored to their needs.

Implement Coping Strategies: Teach your child coping strategies to manage their emotions and mood fluctuations. Help them identify triggers and develop effective techniques to regulate their emotions. This may include deep breathing exercises, mindfulness practices, or engaging in enjoyable activities that provide a sense of calm and balance.

Provide a Safe Outlet: Encourage your child to express their emotions in healthy ways. Offer a safe outlet for them to talk about their experiences, frustrations, and concerns. This may include journaling, drawing, or engaging in creative pursuits that allow them to process their emotions. Supportive discussions and validation of their feelings can help reduce stress and promote emotional well, being.

Encourage Peer Support: Encourage your child to engage in peer support groups or activities that connect them with other young individuals who have bipolar disorder. Peer support can provide a sense of belonging, reduce feelings of isolation, and offer valuable insights and coping strategies. Supportive friendships with peers who understand their experiences can be a source of strength and comfort.

Foster Sibling Understanding: Siblings of children with bipolar disorder may require additional support and understanding. Educate them about bipolar disorder, its impact on their sibling, and how they can contribute to their sibling's well, being. Encourage open communication, empathy, and inclusiveness within the family to ensure a supportive environment for all family members.

Self, Care for Parents: Caring for a child with bipolar disorder can be emotionally demanding. Remember to prioritize your own self, care to maintain your well, being. Seek support from other parents, join support groups, or engage in activities that recharge you.

Chapter Ten

Bipolar Disorder and the Workplace

Bipolar Disorder and the Workplace: Navigating Challenges and Fostering Success

Bipolar disorder, a mental health condition characterized by extreme mood swings, can significantly impact an individual's ability to function in the workplace. However, with the right strategies and support, individuals with bipolar disorder can effectively manage their symptoms, maintain employment, and thrive in their professional lives. By fostering understanding, implementing accommodations, and prioritizing self, care, both employees and employers can create an inclusive and supportive work environment.

Understanding Bipolar Disorder: It is essential for both employees and employers to have a basic understanding of bipolar disorder. Educating oneself about the condition, its symptoms, and its impact on daily functioning promotes empathy, reduces stigma, and fosters a supportive work culture. Recognizing that bipolar disorder is a medical condition and not a character flaw is a crucial first step in creating an inclusive workplace.

Open and Confidential Communication: Encouraging open communication between employees and employers is essential for effectively managing bipolar disorder in the workplace. Employees should feel comfortable disclosing their condition to their employers, either voluntarily or through the appropriate human resources channels. Providing a confidential environment where individuals can discuss their needs, concerns, and potential accommodations promotes trust and enables employers to provide appropriate support.

Accommodations and Flexibility: Implementing workplace accommodations and fostering flexibility can greatly benefit employees with bipolar disorder. Accommodations may include flexible work hours, modified schedules, or the ability to work remotely during periods of increased symptoms or treatment adjustments. Allowing for regular breaks, providing a quiet workspace, or assigning manageable workloads during challenging periods can also support employees in managing their condition effectively.

Job Crafting and Task Management: Job crafting involves tailoring job responsibilities to an employee's strengths, preferences, and capabilities. Collaborating with employees to modify their roles, assign tasks that align with their skills, and minimize triggers can enhance job satisfaction and productivity. Implementing effective task management strategies, such as breaking down projects into smaller, manageable tasks or utilizing project management tools, can help individuals with bipolar disorder maintain focus and reduce stress.

Supportive Work Environment: Creating a supportive work environment is vital for individuals with bipolar disorder. Encouraging a workplace culture that values well, being, mental health, and work, life balance can positively impact employee morale and productivity. Employers can provide resources, such as mental health workshops, training sessions, or access to employee assistance programs (EAPs), to support employees' mental health needs.

Self, Care and Stress Management: Prioritizing self, care is crucial for individuals with bipolar disorder in the workplace. Encouraging employees to engage in self, care activities, such as taking regular breaks, practicing mindfulness, or participating in stress, reducing exercises, promotes overall well, being and resilience. Providing designated spaces for relaxation or promoting wellness programs can also contribute to a healthier work environment.

Employee Assistance Programs (EAPs): Employee Assistance Programs offer confidential support and resources for employees facing personal challenges, including mental health concerns. Employers can ensure that EAPs offer comprehensive mental health services, access to mental health professionals, and referrals for appropriate treatment. Promoting the availability of EAPs and ensuring confidentiality can encourage employees to seek help and support when needed.

Continuity of Treatment: Employers can support employees with bipolar disorder by recognizing the importance of continuity in their treatment. This may involve providing flexibility for medical appointments or accommodating treatment, related needs, such as medication management or therapy sessions. Collaboration between employees, employers, and healthcare providers can ensure that employees receive the necessary support for maintaining their mental health and well, being.

Navigating disclosure and accommodations

Navigating Disclosure and Accommodations: Empowering Individuals with Bipolar Disorder in the Workplace

Disclosure and accommodations are essential considerations for individuals with bipolar disorder in the workplace. Deciding whether or not to disclose a mental health condition and navigating the process of obtaining workplace accommodations can be complex. By understanding the benefits, challenges, and legal rights associated with disclosure, individuals with bipolar disorder can make informed decisions and access the support they need to thrive in their professional lives.

The Decision to Disclose: Disclosure of a mental health condition like bipolar disorder is a personal choice. It is important for individuals to consider the potential benefits and drawbacks before making a decision. Some potential benefits of disclosure include access to workplace accommodations, understanding and support from colleagues and supervisors, and reduced stigma surrounding mental health. However, individuals may also face potential challenges, such as discrimination or prejudice, if their condition is not understood or accepted in the workplace.

Knowing Your Rights: Individuals with bipolar disorder are protected by various laws and regulations that prohibit discrimination in the workplace based on a mental health condition. In many countries, including the United States, the Americans with Disabilities Act (ADA) and the Rehabilitation Act of 1973 provide legal protection against discrimination and require employers to provide reasonable accommodations for individuals with disabilities, including mental health conditions. Familiarize yourself with the laws and regulations applicable to your country to understand your rights and protections.

Timing and Context: The decision to disclose should be carefully considered in terms of timing and context. Assess the workplace culture, relationships with supervisors and colleagues, and the potential impact on your job responsibilities. It may be helpful to disclose when symptoms start to interfere with work or when accommodations are needed. Choosing the right time and context can increase the likelihood of a positive and supportive response from employers and colleagues.

Disclosure Process: If an individual decides to disclose their bipolar disorder, it is important to plan and prepare for the conversation. Choose a private and comfortable setting to discuss the matter with a supervisor, human resources representative, or other appropriate personnel. Provide information about bipolar disorder, its impact on work, and specific accommodations that would be beneficial. Emphasize your commitment to job performance and highlight any successes or coping strategies you have implemented. Maintaining a professional and constructive tone can help facilitate a productive conversation.

Workplace Accommodations: Workplace accommodations are adjustments made to the work environment or job responsibilities that enable individuals with bipolar disorder to perform their duties effectively. Accommodations may include flexible work hours, modified deadlines, reduced workload during periods of high stress, or providing a quiet workspace. The specific accommodations should be tailored to the individual's needs and determined through a collaborative process involving the employee, human resources, and, if necessary, medical professionals. Clear communication and documentation of accommodations are crucial to ensure their implementation.

Requesting Accommodations: When requesting workplace accommodations, it is important to provide clear and detailed information about how the accommodations will support your ability to perform job duties. Prepare a written request outlining the specific accommodations needed and how they relate to the impact of bipolar disorder on your work. Providing documentation from healthcare professionals, such as a doctor's note or a letter outlining recommended accommodations, can strengthen your request. Open communication and collaboration with your employer can help ensure that appropriate accommodations are put in place.

Confidentiality and Privacy: Disclosing a mental health condition does not mean that an individual is required to disclose every detail of their diagnosis or treatment. Employees have the right to privacy and confidentiality regarding their medical information. Information shared during the disclosure process should be kept confidential, shared only with relevant parties who need to be aware of the accommodation process.

Managing job stress and maintaining productivity

Managing Job Stress and Maintaining Productivity: Strategies for Individuals with Bipolar Disorder

Job stress can affect individuals in any profession, but for individuals with bipolar disorder, managing stress is particularly crucial. Bipolar disorder can make individuals more vulnerable to stress, potentially triggering mood episodes and interfering with job performance. However, by implementing effective stress management techniques and prioritizing self, care, individuals with bipolar disorder can navigate job stress and maintain productivity in the workplace.

Recognize Early Warning Signs: Being aware of early warning signs is crucial for managing job stress. Pay attention to changes in mood, sleep patterns, energy levels, and overall well, being. By recognizing early signs of stress, individuals can take proactive steps to manage their symptoms before they escalate.

Establish a Routine: Creating a structured routine can provide stability and reduce stress. Establish consistent work hours, breaks, and daily tasks. Incorporate self, care activities, such as exercise, meditation, or hobbies, into your routine to promote overall well, being and balance.

Prioritize Self, Care: Self, care is essential for managing job stress and maintaining overall mental health. Engage in activities that promote relaxation, such as spending time in nature, practicing mindfulness, or participating in creative outlets. Set aside dedicated time for self, care activities, even during busy workdays, to recharge and reduce stress.

Effective Time Management: Effective time management is crucial for individuals with bipolar disorder. Break down tasks into smaller, manageable steps and prioritize them based on urgency and importance. Utilize tools such as calendars, to, do lists, or project management apps to stay organized and ensure deadlines are met.

Set Boundaries: Setting boundaries in the workplace is important for managing job stress. Learn to say no when necessary and communicate your limitations to supervisors and colleagues. Establishing clear boundaries helps prevent overwhelm and ensures that workloads remain manageable.

Practice Stress, Reduction Techniques: Implementing stress, reduction techniques can significantly alleviate job, related stress. Deep breathing exercises, progressive muscle relaxation, or mindfulness meditation can help reduce anxiety and promote relaxation. Take short breaks throughout the workday to engage in these techniques, allowing for moments of calm and rejuvenation.

Seek Support: It is crucial to build a support network within the workplace. Share concerns, challenges, and successes with trusted colleagues or supervisors who can provide understanding and support. Consider joining support groups outside of work, where you can connect with individuals who share similar experiences and gain insights into managing job stress.

Utilize Accommodations: Workplace accommodations can play a vital role in managing job stress for individuals with bipolar disorder. If you have disclosed your condition, work with your employer to identify and implement appropriate accommodations. This may include flexible work hours, reduced workload during challenging periods, or adjustments to the physical work environment.

Manage Work, Life Balance: Maintaining a healthy work, life balance is crucial for managing job stress. Create boundaries between work and personal life, ensuring that leisure time, family time, and self, care activities are prioritized. Engaging in activities outside of work can help recharge and reduce job, related stress.

Communicate Effectively: Effective communication is key to managing job stress. If you are feeling overwhelmed or experiencing difficulties, communicate with your supervisor or human resources department. Share your needs, concerns, or potential adjustments that could support your job performance. Open communication fosters understanding and allows for collaborative problem, solving.

Take Advantage of Employee Assistance Programs (EAPs): Employee Assistance Programs can provide valuable support for managing job stress. EAPs often offer counseling services, referrals to mental health professionals, and resources for stress management techniques. Take advantage of these programs to access additional support and guidance.

Legal rights and protections

Legal Rights and Protections: Empowering Individuals with Bipolar Disorder in the Workplace

Individuals with bipolar disorder are entitled to legal rights and protections in the workplace. These rights aim to ensure equal opportunities, prevent discrimination, and provide accommodations for individuals with mental health conditions. By understanding these legal provisions, individuals with bipolar disorder can advocate for themselves, address workplace challenges, and access the support they need to thrive professionally.

Americans with Disabilities Act (ADA): In the United States, the Americans with Disabilities Act (ADA) prohibits discrimination against individuals with disabilities, including mental health conditions such as bipolar disorder. Under the ADA, employers with 15 or more employees must provide reasonable accommodations to qualified individuals with disabilities, unless doing so would cause significant difficulty or expense for the employer. Bipolar disorder is recognized as a covered disability under the ADA.

Rehabilitation Act of 1973: The Rehabilitation Act of 1973 is another U.S. law that protects individuals with disabilities, including those with bipolar disorder, in federal employment, government programs, and activities receiving federal financial assistance. Section 504 of the Rehabilitation Act requires employers to provide reasonable accommodations to qualified individuals with disabilities, similar to the ADA.

Reasonable Accommodations: Reasonable accommodations are modifications or adjustments made in the workplace to enable individuals with disabilities to perform their job duties effectively. These accommodations should be tailored to the specific needs of the individual with bipolar disorder. Examples of reasonable accommodations may include flexible work hours, modified deadlines, adjustments to workload or job responsibilities during mood episodes, or modifications to the physical work environment.

Disclosure of Bipolar Disorder: Disclosure of bipolar disorder in the workplace is a personal decision. While some individuals may choose to disclose their condition to their employer or supervisor, others may prefer to keep it confidential. The decision to disclose should be based on individual circumstances, workplace culture, and the potential need for accommodations. Employers cannot require employees to disclose their bipolar disorder, but disclosure may be necessary to access certain protections and accommodations.

Confidentiality and Privacy: Employers are legally obligated to maintain the confidentiality of medical information disclosed by employees, including information related to bipolar disorder. Employers should limit access to this information to those who need it to implement accommodations. Discussing an employee's bipolar disorder or sharing medical information without consent is a violation of privacy rights and can lead to legal consequences.

Prohibition of Discrimination: Employers are prohibited from discriminating against individuals with bipolar disorder. Discrimination can take various forms, including adverse employment actions, such as termination, demotion, or denial of promotion, based on the individual's bipolar disorder. Employers cannot treat employees less favorably due to their condition and must provide equal employment opportunities.

Interactive Process: The interactive process refers to the communication and collaboration between the employer and employee to determine appropriate accommodations. Once an employee discloses their bipolar disorder or requests accommodations, employers must engage in an interactive process to assess the employee's needs and identify suitable accommodations. This process may involve discussing potential accommodations, reviewing medical documentation, and finding solutions that meet both the employee's needs and the employer's operational requirements.

Documentation and Medical Certifications: Employers may request medical documentation or certifications to verify an employee's need for accommodations. Medical documentation should be limited to verifying the existence of a disability and the need for specific accommodations. Employers should not request unnecessary or invasive medical information beyond what is relevant to implementing accommodations.

Retaliation Protection: Employees with bipolar disorder are protected against retaliation for asserting their rights or requesting accommodations. Retaliation can include any adverse employment action, such as harassment, demotion, or termination, taken in response to an employee's exercise of their legal rights.

Chapter Eleven

Bipolar Disorder and Substance Abuse

Bipolar Disorder and Substance Abuse: Understanding the Connection and Seeking Dual Diagnosis Treatment

Bipolar disorder and substance abuse often coexist, creating a complex and challenging situation for individuals affected by both conditions. Bipolar disorder, a mental health condition characterized by extreme mood swings, can increase the risk of developing substance abuse issues. Conversely, substance abuse can exacerbate the symptoms of bipolar disorder and impede effective treatment. Understanding the connection between bipolar disorder and substance abuse and seeking dual diagnosis treatment are crucial steps towards recovery and improved quality of life.

The Connection between Bipolar Disorder and Substance Abuse: There is a strong link between bipolar disorder and substance abuse. Several factors contribute to this connection. Firstly, individuals with bipolar disorder may turn to drugs or alcohol as a means of self, medication, attempting to alleviate the distressing symptoms of their condition. Substance use may temporarily relieve feelings of depression, anxiety, or manic episodes, leading to a cycle of dependence. Additionally, the impulsivity and risk, taking behavior associated with bipolar disorder may increase the likelihood of experimenting with drugs or alcohol.

Substance Abuse Exacerbating Bipolar Symptoms: Substance abuse can exacerbate the symptoms of bipolar disorder and complicate its management. Drug or alcohol use can disrupt the delicate balance of brain chemistry, triggering mood swings and intensifying depressive or manic episodes. Substance abuse may also interfere with medication efficacy, rendering bipolar disorder treatment less effective. Moreover, substances like stimulants or depressants can induce mood fluctuations, making it difficult to differentiate between bipolar symptoms and substance, induced effects.

Dual Diagnosis: Dual diagnosis refers to the coexistence of a mental health disorder, such as bipolar disorder, and substance abuse or addiction. Dual diagnosis is complex and requires an integrated approach to treatment. It is crucial to address both conditions simultaneously to achieve sustainable recovery. Dual diagnosis treatment involves a comprehensive assessment, integrated therapies, and coordinated care by a multidisciplinary team that includes mental health professionals and addiction specialists.

Integrated Treatment Approach: Treating bipolar disorder and substance abuse concurrently requires an integrated treatment approach. Integrated treatment combines therapy, medication management, and substance abuse interventions to address both conditions effectively. Therapeutic modalities such as Cognitive, Behavioral Therapy (CBT), Dialectical Behavior Therapy (DBT), and Motivational Interviewing (MI) are commonly utilized in dual diagnosis treatment. These therapies help individuals develop coping skills, manage cravings, and address underlying psychological issues.

Medication Management: Medication plays a crucial role in managing bipolar disorder, and it is equally important in dual diagnosis treatment. Mood stabilizers, antidepressants, and antipsychotic medications may be prescribed to stabilize mood and manage symptoms of bipolar disorder. In cases of substance abuse, medications like naltrexone or acamprosate can assist in reducing cravings and supporting recovery. Close monitoring by a healthcare professional is necessary to ensure medication adherence and evaluate any potential interactions between psychiatric medications and substances.

Detoxification and Withdrawal Management: For individuals with co, occurring bipolar disorder and substance abuse, a safe and supportive detoxification process may be necessary. Detoxification involves the removal of substances from the body and managing withdrawal symptoms. In a dual diagnosis setting, it is essential to have a comprehensive plan that addresses the specific needs and challenges associated with both bipolar disorder and substance abuse.

Psychoeducation and Skills Building: Psychoeducation is a critical component of dual diagnosis treatment. Individuals with bipolar disorder and substance abuse benefit from understanding the relationship between the two conditions, as well as learning about triggers, coping mechanisms, and relapse prevention strategies. Psychoeducation equips individuals with knowledge and skills to manage their conditions effectively and make informed choices regarding substance use.

Prevalence and risk factors

Prevalence and Risk Factors: Understanding the Landscape of Bipolar Disorders

Bipolar disorder, a complex mental health condition characterized by extreme mood swings, affects millions of people worldwide. Understanding the prevalence and risk factors associated with bipolar disorder is essential for early detection, intervention, and effective management. By exploring the prevalence rates and identifying the various risk factors, we can gain valuable insights into the scope of bipolar disorders and work towards promoting mental health and well, being.

Prevalence of Bipolar Disorders: Bipolar disorder is a relatively common mental health condition, with a significant impact on individuals and society as a whole. The prevalence rates vary across populations and studies, but estimates suggest that approximately 1, 3% of the global population experiences bipolar disorder at some point in their lives. It affects people of all genders, ages, and ethnic backgrounds, indicating that no specific demographic group is immune to its impact.

Age of Onset: Bipolar disorder can manifest at any age, but it often emerges during late adolescence or early adulthood. Research suggests that the average age of onset is around 25 years, although some individuals may experience symptoms earlier or later in life. It is essential to recognize the signs and symptoms of bipolar disorder during adolescence and provide appropriate support and intervention.

Gender Differences: Bipolar disorder affects both males and females, but some gender differences exist in terms of prevalence and symptom presentation. Studies indicate that females are more likely to experience rapid cycling (frequent mood shifts) and depressive episodes, while males may be more prone to experiencing manic episodes. However, it is important to note that these gender differences may vary, and individual experiences can differ significantly.

Genetic Factors: Genetic predisposition plays a significant role in the development of bipolar disorder. Family and twin studies have consistently shown that individuals with a first, degree relative (parent, sibling, or child) with bipolar disorder are at higher risk of developing the condition themselves. However, genetic factors alone do not fully explain the development of bipolar disorder, suggesting that other environmental and biological factors also contribute to its onset.

Biological and Neurochemical Factors: Imbalances in brain chemicals (neurotransmitters) and irregularities in brain structures and circuits are thought to be involved in bipolar disorder. Research has highlighted abnormalities in the levels of neurotransmitters such as serotonin, dopamine, and norepinephrine, which regulate mood and emotions. Structural and functional brain imaging studies have also identified differences in specific brain regions, further supporting the role of biological factors in the development of bipolar disorder.

Environmental Factors: Environmental factors can interact with genetic and biological factors to increase the risk of developing bipolar disorder. Traumatic life events, such as abuse, neglect, or significant loss, can contribute to the onset or exacerbation of bipolar symptoms. Chronic stress, substance abuse, sleep disturbances, and disruptions in circadian rhythms have also been associated with an increased risk of bipolar disorder. These factors can trigger or worsen mood episodes and contribute to the overall course of the disorder.

Substance Abuse and Bipolar Disorder: Substance abuse and bipolar disorder often coexist, creating a complex and challenging situation for individuals affected by both conditions. Substance abuse, particularly alcohol and illicit drugs, can worsen the symptoms of bipolar disorder, increase the frequency of mood episodes, and interfere with treatment efficacy. Conversely, individuals with bipolar disorder may turn to substance abuse as a form of self, medication, attempting to alleviate the distressing symptoms of their condition.

Dual diagnosis treatment approaches

Dual Diagnosis Treatment Approaches: Addressing Co, Occurring Bipolar Disorder and Substance Abuse

Dual diagnosis refers to the coexistence of a mental health disorder, such as bipolar disorder, and substance abuse or addiction. Individuals with dual diagnoses face unique challenges that require specialized treatment approaches. Effective dual diagnosis treatment recognizes the interplay between bipolar disorder and substance abuse, and it integrates interventions to address both conditions concurrently. By understanding the principles and approaches of dual diagnosis treatment, individuals can receive comprehensive care and improve their chances of sustained recovery.

Integrated Treatment: Integrated treatment is the cornerstone of dual diagnosis care. It involves a comprehensive and coordinated approach that addresses both bipolar disorder and substance abuse simultaneously. Rather than treating these conditions separately, integrated treatment recognizes their interrelationship and the impact each has on the other. Integrated treatment plans are tailored to meet the individual's specific needs and may include a combination of pharmacotherapy, psychotherapy, and support services.

Comprehensive Assessment: A thorough assessment is crucial in dual diagnosis treatment to understand the individual's unique needs and determine the severity of both conditions. This assessment involves evaluating psychiatric symptoms, substance abuse patterns, medical history, social factors, and any co, occurring disorders. The information gathered during the assessment guides the development of an individualized treatment plan.

Pharmacotherapy: Medication management is an essential component of dual diagnosis treatment. Psychiatric medications, such as mood stabilizers, antipsychotics, and antidepressants, are commonly prescribed to manage the symptoms of bipolar disorder. Medications for substance abuse, such as those that reduce cravings or alleviate withdrawal symptoms, may also be incorporated into the treatment plan. Close monitoring by healthcare professionals is necessary to assess medication effectiveness and address any potential interactions or side effects.

Psychotherapy: Psychotherapy plays a critical role in dual diagnosis treatment, helping individuals address the underlying factors contributing to both bipolar disorder and substance abuse. Various therapeutic modalities can be effective, including Cognitive, Behavioral Therapy (CBT), Dialectical Behavior Therapy (DBT), and Motivational Interviewing (MI). These therapies assist individuals in developing coping skills, managing cravings, improving mood regulation, and enhancing motivation for change.

Relapse Prevention: Relapse prevention strategies are essential in dual diagnosis treatment. Substance abuse and bipolar disorder can both present challenges that may lead to relapse. By identifying triggers, developing coping mechanisms, and learning skills for managing cravings and mood fluctuations, individuals can better navigate the challenges of recovery. Relapse prevention strategies may include developing a support network, creating a relapse prevention plan, and learning healthy coping mechanisms to manage stress and emotions.

Supportive Group Therapy: Group therapy provides a valuable forum for individuals to connect with peers who share similar experiences. Supportive group therapy can help individuals with dual diagnoses develop a sense of belonging, reduce feelings of isolation, and gain insight from others who have faced similar challenges. Group therapy also provides an opportunity for individuals to practice interpersonal skills, receive support, and learn from the successes and setbacks of their peers.

Psychoeducation: Psychoeducation plays a crucial role in dual diagnosis treatment by providing individuals with information about bipolar disorder, substance abuse, and the relationship between the two. Understanding the underlying mechanisms, triggers, and consequences of both conditions empowers individuals to take an active role in their treatment. Psychoeducation sessions can cover topics such as medication management, coping strategies, relapse prevention, and healthy lifestyle choices.

Strategies for maintaining sobriety

Strategies for Maintaining Sobriety: Navigating Recovery with Bipolar Disorder

Maintaining sobriety is a challenging but essential goal for individuals with bipolar disorder and co, occurring substance abuse. Bipolar disorder can complicate the recovery process, as mood fluctuations and impulsivity can increase the risk of relapse. However, by implementing effective strategies and adopting a comprehensive approach, individuals can navigate the journey of recovery, manage their bipolar symptoms, and maintain long, term sobriety.

Build a Supportive Network: Surrounding oneself with a supportive network is crucial for maintaining sobriety. Connect with individuals who understand the challenges of both bipolar disorder and substance abuse. This may involve attending support groups, such as Dual Recovery Anonymous or Alcoholics Anonymous, where individuals share their experiences and provide encouragement. Engaging in therapy or counseling can also provide valuable support and guidance.

Create a Relapse Prevention Plan: Developing a relapse prevention plan is essential for individuals in recovery. This plan includes identifying triggers, developing coping strategies, and establishing healthy habits. Recognize the warning signs of a potential relapse, such as changes in mood, increased stress, or social isolation. Implement strategies to address these warning signs proactively, such as engaging in healthy activities, seeking support, and practicing self, care.

Prioritize Self, Care: Self, care is crucial for maintaining sobriety and managing bipolar disorder. Prioritize activities that promote physical, emotional, and mental well, being. Engage in regular exercise, practice relaxation techniques, and ensure adequate sleep. Establish healthy eating habits and avoid substances that can destabilize mood, such as caffeine or excessive sugar. Taking care of oneself holistically can strengthen resilience and contribute to overall stability.

Manage Stress Effectively: Stress can be a significant trigger for both bipolar symptoms and substance abuse cravings. Develop effective stress management techniques to reduce the risk of relapse. Explore various stress, reduction strategies, such as mindfulness meditation, deep breathing exercises, or engaging in hobbies that promote relaxation. Create a healthy work, life balance and set boundaries to minimize stressors in daily life.

Engage in Dual Diagnosis Treatment: Dual diagnosis treatment addresses both bipolar disorder and substance abuse concurrently. Engaging in specialized treatment programs that cater to individuals with co, occurring disorders is essential. Dual diagnosis treatment provides comprehensive care, integrating therapy, medication management, and support services to address both conditions effectively. Seek professional help from providers experienced in treating dual diagnosis to ensure a holistic and tailored approach to recovery.

Monitor Medication and Treatment: Medication adherence and ongoing treatment for bipolar disorder are critical for maintaining sobriety. Work closely with healthcare professionals to ensure that medication is taken as prescribed and to monitor its effectiveness. Attend regular therapy sessions to address underlying issues, develop coping strategies, and receive ongoing support. Open communication with treatment providers is vital to manage bipolar symptoms effectively and prevent relapse.

Practice Mindfulness and Emotional Regulation: Bipolar disorder can bring intense emotions and mood swings. Developing mindfulness practices and emotional regulation techniques can help manage these fluctuations and reduce the risk of turning to substances as a means of coping. Engage in mindfulness meditation, which can enhance self, awareness and provide a sense of grounding. Learn healthy ways to identify, express, and regulate emotions to avoid impulsive behaviors.

Identify and Address Co, Occurring Issues: Individuals with bipolar disorder and substance abuse may have underlying issues, such as trauma, anxiety, or low self, esteem, that contribute to their conditions. Identifying and addressing these co, occurring issues is crucial for maintaining sobriety. Engage in therapy or counseling to explore these underlying concerns and develop healthier coping mechanisms. Targeting the root causes of substance abuse can promote lasting recovery.

Chapter Twelve

Bipolar Disorder and Suicide Prevention

Bipolar Disorder and Suicide Prevention: Promoting Awareness and Support

Bipolar disorder is a complex mental health condition characterized by extreme mood swings that can significantly impact an individual's well, being. One of the most concerning aspects of bipolar disorder is the increased risk of suicide. Understanding the connection between bipolar disorder and suicide, recognizing warning signs, and implementing preventive strategies are crucial for promoting mental health and saving lives.

The Link Between Bipolar Disorder and Suicide: Individuals with bipolar disorder face a higher risk of suicidal thoughts and behaviors compared to the general population. The intense mood swings and emotional dysregulation associated with bipolar disorder can contribute to feelings of despair, hopelessness, and impulsivity. It is estimated that up to 20% of individuals with bipolar disorder attempt suicide at least once in their lifetime. Suicide prevention efforts within the context of bipolar disorder are of utmost importance.

Recognizing Warning Signs: Recognizing warning signs is vital for identifying individuals at risk of suicide. While it is essential to remember that not all individuals will exhibit warning signs, some common indicators include:

a. Expressing feelings of hopelessness, worthlessness, or being a burden to others.

b. Withdrawing from social interactions and isolating oneself.

c. Increased frequency or intensity of depressive or manic symptoms.

d. Talking about death, dying, or suicide, even in a vague or indirect manner.

e. Giving away belongings or making final arrangements.

f. Engaging in reckless behaviors or displaying sudden calmness after a period of intense mood swings.

Seeking Professional Help: Encouraging individuals with bipolar disorder to seek professional help is crucial for suicide prevention. Mental health professionals, such as psychiatrists, psychologists, or licensed therapists, can provide comprehensive assessments, diagnosis, and evidence, based treatments. The combination of medication management and psychotherapy, including Cognitive, Behavioral Therapy (CBT), can significantly reduce the risk of suicide by addressing underlying issues and providing coping strategies.

Developing a Safety Plan: A safety plan is a personalized set of strategies that individuals can use when they experience suicidal thoughts or are in crisis. Collaborating with mental health professionals, individuals can develop a safety plan that includes coping mechanisms, emergency contacts, and a list of supportive resources. Having a safety plan in place empowers individuals to take proactive steps in managing their mental health and seeking assistance when needed.

Creating a Supportive Environment: Creating a supportive environment is essential for suicide prevention among individuals with bipolar disorder.

Loved ones, friends, and colleagues can play a crucial role in promoting mental health and providing support. Active listening, empathy, and non, judgmental attitudes can help individuals feel understood and valued. Encourage open communication, validate their experiences, and offer assistance in seeking professional help.

Education and Psychoeducation: Education about bipolar disorder and suicide prevention is key to increasing awareness and reducing stigma. Providing accurate information about the condition, its symptoms, and the link to suicide can help individuals understand their experiences and seek appropriate help. Psychoeducation programs, support groups, and community workshops can offer valuable insights into managing bipolar disorder and fostering mental wellness.

Enhancing Coping Skills: Developing effective coping skills is essential for individuals with bipolar disorder to manage emotional challenges and reduce suicide risk. Coping mechanisms may include engaging in regular exercise, practicing relaxation techniques, maintaining a healthy lifestyle, expressing emotions through creative outlets, and seeking social support. Encourage individuals to identify healthy coping strategies that work best for them and integrate them into their daily lives.

Warning signs and risk factors

Warning Signs and Risk Factors: Identifying the Red Flags of Bipolar Disorders

Bipolar disorder is a complex mental health condition characterized by extreme mood swings that can significantly impact an individual's well, being. Recognizing the warning signs and understanding the risk factors associated with bipolar disorders are crucial for early detection, intervention, and effective management. By familiarizing ourselves with the red flags and risk factors, we can promote mental health awareness and provide support to those in need.

Persistent Mood Swings: Mood swings are a hallmark of bipolar disorder. Individuals with bipolar disorder experience distinct periods of mania or hypomania, characterized by elevated mood, increased energy, racing thoughts, and impulsivity. These periods are followed by depressive episodes, characterized by sadness, loss of interest, low energy, and feelings of hopelessness. Recognizing significant and persistent mood swings beyond the normal ups and downs of life is essential in identifying potential bipolar disorder.

Changes in Energy and Sleep Patterns: Individuals with bipolar disorder often experience drastic changes in energy levels and sleep patterns. During manic or hypomanic episodes, individuals may exhibit an increased need for sleep or a decreased need for sleep, feeling energized and functioning with little rest. Conversely, during depressive episodes, individuals may experience excessive fatigue and an increased need for sleep, struggling to maintain their usual energy levels.

Impaired Judgment and Risky Behavior: Impaired judgment and engaging in risky behavior are common symptoms of bipolar disorder during manic or hypomanic episodes. Individuals may exhibit impulsive actions such as excessive spending, engaging in reckless sexual behavior, substance abuse, or pursuing grandiose plans without considering the consequences. Recognizing these behaviors as more than occasional impulsivity can be crucial in identifying potential bipolar disorder.

Changes in Appetite and Weight: Bipolar disorder can influence appetite and weight. During depressive episodes, individuals may experience a loss of appetite, resulting in weight loss. Conversely, during manic or hypomanic episodes, individuals may have an increased appetite, leading to weight gain. Significant and unexplained changes in appetite and weight that are not attributable to other factors should be considered potential warning signs of bipolar disorder.

Difficulty Concentrating and Making Decisions: Cognitive impairments, such as difficulty concentrating, making decisions, or experiencing memory problems, are common symptoms during both manic and depressive episodes. Individuals may struggle to focus on tasks, experience a decline in work or academic performance, or find it challenging to retain information. These cognitive impairments can significantly impact daily functioning and should be considered potential indicators of bipolar disorder.

Social Withdrawal and Isolation: Bipolar disorder can lead to social withdrawal and isolation, particularly during depressive episodes. Individuals may lose interest in activities they once enjoyed, withdraw from social interactions, and isolate themselves from friends and family. Recognizing significant changes in social behavior and the absence of interest in previously enjoyed activities can be crucial in identifying potential bipolar disorder.

Suicidal Thoughts or Behaviors: Bipolar disorder is associated with an increased risk of suicidal thoughts and behaviors. Individuals may express feelings of hopelessness, express a desire to die, or exhibit self, harming behaviors. It is essential to take any mention of suicide seriously and seek immediate professional help if an individual expresses suicidal thoughts or engages in self, harm.

Family History of Bipolar Disorder: Having a family history of bipolar disorder significantly increases the risk of developing the condition. If a close family member, such as a parent or sibling, has been diagnosed with bipolar disorder, it is important to be aware of the potential risk and monitor for any signs or symptoms that may indicate the presence of the disorder.

Traumatic Life Events: Traumatic life events, such as abuse, neglect, significant loss, or major life transitions, can increase the risk of developing bipolar disorders.

Crisis intervention and safety planning

Crisis Intervention and Safety Planning: Supporting Individuals with Bipolar Disorders

Bipolar disorder is a complex mental health condition characterized by extreme mood swings that can significantly impact an individual's well, being. During times of crisis or heightened symptoms, individuals with bipolar disorder may require immediate intervention and support. Crisis intervention and safety planning play a crucial role in providing immediate assistance, promoting stability, and ensuring the safety of individuals experiencing bipolar crises.

Recognizing a Crisis: It is important to be able to identify when an individual with bipolar disorder is experiencing a crisis. A crisis can manifest as a severe depressive episode, an intense manic or hypomanic episode, or an acute suicidal or self, harming episode. Common signs may include extreme changes in mood, impaired judgment, heightened agitation, expressions of hopelessness, or threats of self, harm. Recognizing these signs can help prompt appropriate intervention.

Stay Calm and Provide Reassurance: When assisting someone in crisis, it is crucial to remain calm and composed. Reassure the individual that they are not alone and that help is available. Maintain a non, judgmental and empathetic attitude, emphasizing your willingness to listen and support them. Your calm demeanor can help create a safe and trusting environment for the individual.

Encourage Open Communication: Encouraging open communication is essential during a crisis. Create a safe space for the individual to express their feelings, concerns, and thoughts without fear of judgment. Active listening and empathy are key elements in fostering open communication. Avoid interrupting or dismissing their experiences and validate their emotions.

Contact Emergency Services if Necessary: If the individual's safety is at immediate risk or they express intent to harm themselves or others, it is important to contact emergency services. Provide them with the necessary information, such as the person's name, location, and a brief description of the situation. Emergency services can dispatch appropriate personnel to provide immediate assistance and ensure the safety of the individual.

Involve a Support Network: Crisis intervention should involve the individual's support network, such as family members, friends, or mental health professionals. Contacting a trusted person who is familiar with the individual's condition can provide additional support and assistance during the crisis. Involving mental health professionals, such as psychiatrists or therapists, who are familiar with the individual's treatment plan can help ensure continuity of care.

Implement Safety Planning: Safety planning is a proactive approach that individuals with bipolar disorder can undertake to manage crises and reduce harm. Safety planning involves developing a personalized plan that includes strategies for coping with triggers, identifying supportive individuals to contact in times of crisis, and establishing guidelines for seeking professional help. A safety plan may also include a list of emergency contact numbers, crisis hotlines, and mental health resources.

Remove Access to Means of Self, Harm: During a crisis, it is crucial to identify and remove any potential means of self, harm or suicide. This may involve safely securing objects such as medications, sharp objects, or firearms that could be used to inflict harm. Engaging family members or trusted individuals in the process can help ensure the individual's safety.

Encourage Professional Intervention: Crisis intervention should always be followed by professional intervention. Encourage the individual to seek immediate professional help, whether through their psychiatrist, therapist, or a crisis hotline. Mental health professionals can assess the severity of the crisis, adjust treatment plans if necessary, and provide ongoing support to prevent future crises.

Maintain a Supportive Environment: After the crisis has subsided, it is crucial to maintain a supportive environment for the individual. Check, in regularly, show concern, and continue to encourage open communication. Be patient and understanding, as the recovery process can be challenging.

Postvention and support for survivors

Postvention and Support for Survivors: Healing and Rebuilding Lives Affected by Bipolar Disorders

When a loss occurs due to suicide, the aftermath leaves family members, friends, and the community devastated. Postvention, the term used to describe the support and intervention offered after a suicide, is crucial in helping survivors cope with their grief and rebuild their lives. In the context of bipolar disorders, where the risk of suicide is elevated, providing effective postvention strategies and support is essential in promoting healing, preventing further harm, and fostering resilience among survivors.

Immediate Support and Communication: Immediately following a suicide, it is important to provide immediate support and communicate with the survivors. Reach out to them personally or through designated individuals to express condolences, offer help, and provide information about available resources. Open and honest communication establishes a foundation of support and assures survivors that they are not alone in their grief.

Coordination with Mental Health Professionals: Engage mental health professionals who specialize in grief counseling and trauma to support the survivors. These professionals can provide individual and group counseling, facilitate support groups, and offer guidance on coping strategies. Coordination with mental health professionals ensures survivors receive appropriate care that addresses their specific needs.

Education and Psychoeducation: Educating survivors about suicide, mental health, and bipolar disorder can help dispel misconceptions and reduce stigma. Psychoeducation sessions can provide survivors with a better understanding of the complex nature of bipolar disorders and the challenges faced by individuals with the condition. By promoting education and understanding, survivors can develop empathy and support for those affected by bipolar disorders.

Support Groups: Support groups play a vital role in postvention, offering a safe space for survivors to connect, share experiences, and receive support from others who have gone through similar losses. Support groups provide validation, comfort, and a sense of community, reducing feelings of isolation and fostering healing. Professional facilitation and peer support can guide survivors in navigating the grieving process.

Grief Counseling and Therapy: Grief counseling and therapy are essential components of postvention for survivors. Individual counseling allows survivors to process their grief, explore complex emotions, and develop coping mechanisms. Therapists trained in grief counseling provide a non, judgmental space for survivors to express their feelings and find healthy ways to navigate through their grief journey.

Memorialization and Remembrance: Creating opportunities for survivors to memorialize their loved ones and honor their memory can be a meaningful part of the healing process. Memorial events, such as candlelight vigils, memorial services, or art exhibitions, provide a space for survivors to come together, share stories, and remember their loved ones in a supportive environment. These events can foster a sense of closure and provide an outlet for collective grieving.

Facilitating Social Support: Encourage survivors to lean on their existing support networks, such as family, friends, and faith communities. Facilitating social support involves helping survivors identify individuals who can provide emotional support, practical assistance, or simply a listening ear. Engaging in activities that promote social connectedness can mitigate feelings of loneliness and help survivors rebuild their lives.

Building Resilience: Supporting survivors in building resilience is crucial in postvention. Resilience allows individuals to adapt to adversity, navigate grief, and move forward in life. Encourage survivors to engage in self, care activities, such as exercise, meditation, or creative outlets, that promote emotional well, being. Provide resources and guidance on healthy coping strategies to foster resilience and empower survivors to find strength in their journey of healing.

Promoting Continued Education and Advocacy: Encourage survivors to become advocates for mental health and suicide prevention. By sharing their stories, survivors can raise awareness, reduce stigma, and advocate for improved mental health support and resources.

Chapter Thirteen

Bipolar Disorder and Pregnancy

Bipolar Disorder and Pregnancy: Navigating the Complexities of Mental Health and Maternal Well, being

Pregnancy is a time of significant physical, emotional, and hormonal changes, which can impact women's mental health. For women with bipolar disorder, the complexities are heightened as they navigate the challenges of pregnancy while managing their condition. Understanding the relationship between bipolar disorder and pregnancy, identifying potential risks, and implementing appropriate strategies are essential for promoting maternal well, being and ensuring a healthy pregnancy.

Pregnancy and Bipolar Disorder: Pregnancy can influence the course of bipolar disorder, and bipolar disorder can affect the experience of pregnancy. The hormonal changes during pregnancy may impact mood stability, leading to fluctuations in bipolar symptoms. Additionally, the stress and emotional adjustments associated with pregnancy can pose challenges for women with bipolar disorder. It is important to recognize that each woman's experience will vary, and individualized care is necessary.

Medication Management: Medication management is a critical consideration for pregnant women with bipolar disorder. Some medications used to manage bipolar symptoms may pose potential risks to the developing fetus. It is essential to consult with a healthcare professional experienced in treating pregnant women with bipolar disorder to weigh the benefits and risks of medication use during pregnancy. In some cases, medication adjustments or alternative treatments may be explored to ensure the health of both the mother and the baby.

Careful Planning and Preconception Counseling: Preconception counseling is essential for women with bipolar disorder who are planning to conceive. It involves discussions with healthcare professionals to assess the readiness for pregnancy, review medication management, and develop a plan for managing bipolar symptoms during pregnancy. Planning ahead allows for adjustments in treatment, monitoring of potential risks, and preparation for the unique challenges that may arise.

Close Monitoring and Regular Check, ups: Close monitoring throughout pregnancy is crucial for women with bipolar disorder. Regular prenatal check, ups and mental health evaluations allow healthcare providers to assess the well, being of both the mother and the baby. This monitoring helps identify any changes in bipolar symptoms, assess medication efficacy, and address any potential complications that may arise during pregnancy.

Supportive Care and Therapy: Pregnant women with bipolar disorder can benefit from supportive care and therapy. Engaging in therapy, such as cognitive, behavioral therapy (CBT), can help women develop coping strategies, manage stress, and navigate the emotional changes that accompany pregnancy. Supportive care, including regular check, ins with healthcare professionals, can provide reassurance, education, and guidance throughout the pregnancy journey.

Lifestyle Modifications: Making lifestyle modifications can contribute to the overall well, being of pregnant women with bipolar disorder. Prioritizing self, care, including adequate sleep, regular exercise, and a healthy diet, can support mood stability and physical health. Avoiding substances such as alcohol and recreational drugs is crucial to prevent potential complications and minimize the risk of triggering bipolar episodes.

Establishing a Support System: Building a strong support system is vital for pregnant women with bipolar disorder. This includes involving partners, family members, and friends who can provide emotional support and assistance with daily tasks. Joining support groups or seeking peer support from other women with bipolar disorder who have experienced pregnancy can also provide a sense of community and shared experiences.

Postpartum Care: Postpartum care is an important aspect of managing bipolar disorder after giving birth. The postpartum period poses unique challenges, including hormonal changes, sleep deprivation, and the adjustment to new motherhood. Establishing a postpartum care plan that includes regular check, ins with healthcare professionals, support from loved ones, and access to mental health resources is crucial for promoting a smooth transition into motherhood while managing bipolar disorder.

Planning for pregnancy and managing medications

Planning for Pregnancy and Managing Medications: Navigating the Intersection of Bipolar Disorders and Maternal Health

Planning for pregnancy requires careful consideration and preparation, particularly for women with bipolar disorder. Balancing the management of bipolar symptoms with the potential risks of medication use during pregnancy can present challenges. Understanding the importance of planning, seeking medical guidance, and making informed decisions regarding medication management is essential for women with bipolar disorder who are considering pregnancy. By navigating the complexities of bipolar disorders and maternal health, women can optimize their well, being and ensure a healthy pregnancy.

Preconception Counseling: Preconception counseling is a vital step for women with bipolar disorder who are planning to conceive. It involves consulting with healthcare professionals experienced in managing bipolar disorder during pregnancy. During these discussions, potential risks and benefits of medication use, adjustments in treatment plans, and strategies for managing bipolar symptoms are evaluated. Preconception counseling allows for the development of a personalized plan to ensure the health and well, being of both the mother and the baby.

Timing of Pregnancy: Timing pregnancy with bipolar disorder management is an important consideration. It is generally recommended that women achieve stability in their bipolar symptoms before attempting to conceive. This stability allows for optimal management of the condition during pregnancy. Women should work closely with their healthcare providers to assess their readiness for pregnancy based on their individual circumstances and the severity of their bipolar symptoms.

Medication Evaluation: The use of medication for bipolar disorder management during pregnancy requires careful evaluation. Some medications used to treat bipolar disorder may pose potential risks to the developing fetus. The decision regarding medication use during pregnancy should be made in collaboration with healthcare professionals. The benefits of medication in stabilizing bipolar symptoms must be weighed against the potential risks to the baby. In some cases, medication adjustments or alternative treatments may be explored to ensure maternal well, being and minimize fetal risks.

Risks and Benefits Discussion: When considering medication management during pregnancy, a thorough discussion of the risks and benefits is essential. Healthcare professionals can provide information on the specific medications used, their potential effects on pregnancy, and alternative options. They can also address concerns regarding the impact of medication changes on bipolar symptom management. Open and honest communication is crucial for informed decision, making.

Individualized Treatment Plans: Recognizing that each woman's experience with bipolar disorder is unique, treatment plans should be individualized to meet their specific needs. This includes tailoring medication regimens to achieve the optimal balance between symptom management and minimizing potential risks during pregnancy. Healthcare providers should closely monitor the effectiveness of medications and adjust dosages as necessary, ensuring the health and stability of the mother while considering the well, being of the developing baby.

Risk, Reduction Strategies: In cases where medication adjustments are necessary or when women decide to discontinue medication during pregnancy, risk, reduction strategies should be implemented. These strategies may involve close monitoring of bipolar symptoms, implementing non, pharmacological interventions such as therapy or counseling, and providing additional support during pregnancy. Healthcare providers can guide women in developing coping mechanisms and alternative strategies to manage bipolar symptoms during this period.

Multidisciplinary Collaboration: Managing bipolar disorder during pregnancy requires a multidisciplinary approach. Collaboration among healthcare professionals, including psychiatrists, obstetricians, and primary care physicians, is crucial for effective management. Regular communication ensures coordinated care, providing a holistic approach to maternal well, being and fetal health.

Emotional Support and Therapy: Pregnancy can be emotionally challenging for women with bipolar disorder. Emotional support and therapy play important roles in managing mental health during this period. Therapy sessions can help women develop coping mechanisms, enhance self, care strategies, and navigate the emotional changes that accompany pregnancy. Emotional support from loved ones, support groups, or peer networks can also provide valuable reassurance and understanding.

Postpartum mood episodes and support strategies

Postpartum Mood Episodes and Support Strategies: Nurturing Maternal Well, being in the Context of Bipolar Disorders

The postpartum period is a time of immense joy and adjustment for new mothers. However, for women with bipolar disorder, this period may also bring the risk of postpartum mood episodes. Managing bipolar symptoms while caring for a newborn can be challenging, making it crucial to understand postpartum mood episodes and implement effective support strategies. By promoting awareness, providing support, and implementing appropriate interventions, we can nurture maternal well, being and ensure a positive postpartum experience.

Postpartum Mood Episodes: Postpartum mood episodes can occur in women with bipolar disorder, which may include postpartum depression, postpartum mania, or postpartum psychosis. Postpartum depression can present with symptoms such as persistent sadness, loss of interest, changes in appetite, sleep disturbances, and difficulty bonding with the baby. Postpartum mania may involve increased energy, racing thoughts, irritability, and impulsive behavior. Postpartum psychosis is the most severe and rarest form, characterized by hallucinations, delusions, confusion, and disorientation. Recognizing the signs of postpartum mood episodes is crucial for early intervention.

Identifying Risk Factors: Several factors can contribute to the risk of postpartum mood episodes in women with bipolar disorder. These may include a history of postpartum mood episodes, a history of severe bipolar symptoms, inadequate social support, stressful life events, or a lack of effective treatment. Identifying these risk factors can help healthcare professionals and support networks implement targeted strategies to reduce the risk and provide appropriate support.

Medication Management: Medication management is a critical aspect of supporting women with bipolar disorder during the postpartum period. Healthcare providers can assess the safety and effectiveness of medication use while breastfeeding and adjust medication regimens as necessary. For some women, the continuation of medication during the postpartum period may be essential to stabilize mood and prevent mood episodes. Balancing the benefits of medication with potential risks to the baby is a complex decision that requires careful consideration and medical guidance.

Psychoeducation: Psychoeducation is an essential component of postpartum support for women with bipolar disorder. Providing education about postpartum mood episodes, their symptoms, and available treatment options helps women and their families understand and recognize the signs of distress. Psychoeducation empowers individuals to seek timely help, reduce self, blame, and actively engage in their recovery process.

Emotional Support: Emotional support is crucial for women experiencing postpartum mood episodes. Loved ones, family members, and friends can play a significant role in providing a supportive and non, judgmental environment. Active listening, empathy, and understanding can help women feel heard and validated. Encouraging open communication and expressing concern can foster a sense of security and promote help, seeking behaviors.

Supportive Therapy: Engaging in supportive therapy is beneficial for women with bipolar disorder during the postpartum period. Supportive therapy provides a safe space to discuss and process emotions, gain coping skills, and develop strategies for managing postpartum mood episodes. Therapists trained in postpartum mental health can offer guidance on self, care, stress management, and effective communication within relationships.

Support Groups: Support groups specifically tailored to postpartum mood episodes provide a valuable platform for women to connect with others who share similar experiences. Support groups can reduce feelings of isolation and provide a sense of community. Sharing personal stories, coping strategies, and resources can be empowering and reassuring for women navigating postpartum mood episodes.

Parenting with bipolar disorder

Parenting with Bipolar Disorder: Nurturing Families and Managing Bipolar Symptoms

Parenting is a challenging yet rewarding journey, and for individuals with bipolar disorder, it brings unique considerations and responsibilities. Nurturing a family while managing bipolar symptoms requires careful self, care, support systems, and effective strategies. By understanding the impact of bipolar disorder on parenting, implementing coping mechanisms, and seeking support, individuals with bipolar disorder can create a stable and nurturing environment for their children.

Understanding the Impact: Bipolar disorder can influence parenting in various ways. Mood fluctuations may affect the ability to provide consistent emotional support and stability. However, it is important to remember that having bipolar disorder does not automatically make someone a "bad" parent. Recognizing the potential challenges and seeking appropriate support can help individuals navigate their parenting journey effectively.

Self, Care and Stability: Prioritizing self, care is crucial for parents with bipolar disorder. Consistency in self, care routines, such as maintaining a regular sleep schedule, engaging in stress, reducing activities, and taking medication as prescribed, can contribute to mood stability. When parents prioritize their own well, being, they are better equipped to provide a stable and nurturing environment for their children.

Open Communication: Honest and open communication within the family is essential. Age, appropriate discussions about bipolar disorder can help children understand their parent's condition, reduce stigma, and foster empathy. Encouraging children to ask questions and express their feelings in a safe and supportive environment can strengthen family bonds and facilitate understanding.

Creating Predictability and Routine: Establishing predictability and routine within the household can provide stability for both children and parents. Consistent daily schedules, regular meal times, and predictable routines help create a sense of security and structure. By maintaining a stable environment, parents can manage their bipolar symptoms more effectively and promote a sense of calmness within the family.

Seeking Support: Building a support network is crucial for parents with bipolar disorder. Seeking support from family members, friends, or support groups can provide emotional validation, practical assistance, and a sense of belonging. Parenting support groups specifically tailored to individuals with mental health conditions can offer valuable insights, shared experiences, and guidance on managing the challenges of parenting with bipolar disorder.

Co, Parenting and Coping Strategies: Co, parenting with a partner or trusted family member can help distribute the responsibilities of parenting and provide additional support. Developing effective coping strategies, such as engaging in self, soothing techniques, practicing mindfulness, or using relaxation exercises, can help parents manage stress and prevent mood episodes that may impact parenting.

Utilizing Professional Support: Mental health professionals can play a significant role in supporting parents with bipolar disorder. Engaging in therapy or counseling can provide a safe space to discuss parenting challenges, develop coping strategies, and receive guidance on managing bipolar symptoms within the context of parenting. Psychiatrists or healthcare providers can monitor medication effectiveness, adjust treatment plans if necessary, and provide ongoing support.

Modeling Healthy Coping Mechanisms: Parents with bipolar disorder have an opportunity to model healthy coping mechanisms for their children. By practicing self, care, managing stress effectively, and seeking support when needed, parents can demonstrate positive ways of managing their condition. This not only promotes their own well, being but also teaches children important skills for managing challenges in their own lives.

Embracing Flexibility and Self, Compassion: Recognizing that parenting is a journey filled with ups and downs, it is important for parents with bipolar disorder to embrace flexibility and practice self, compassion. Accepting that there may be challenging moments and setbacks allows parents to approach their parenting journey with realistic expectations. Showing kindness and understanding toward oneself fosters resilience and empowers parents to navigate the complexities of parenting with bipolar disorder.

Chapter Fourteen

Stigma and Misconceptions

Stigma and Misconceptions: Breaking Down Barriers in Understanding Bipolar Disorders

Bipolar disorder is a complex mental health condition that affects millions of individuals worldwide. Despite its prevalence, stigma and misconceptions surrounding bipolar disorders persist in society. These misconceptions contribute to discrimination, hinder access to proper treatment, and create barriers to support for individuals with bipolar disorder. By challenging stigma and fostering understanding, we can create a more inclusive and supportive environment for those living with bipolar disorders.

Stigma and its Impact: Stigma refers to the negative attitudes, beliefs, and stereotypes associated with mental health conditions such as bipolar disorder. Stigma creates a climate of fear, judgment, and discrimination, leading to social isolation, diminished self, esteem, and limited opportunities for individuals with bipolar disorder. It can also prevent individuals from seeking help and support, exacerbating the challenges they face.

Dispelling Misconceptions: Education is key to dispelling misconceptions surrounding bipolar disorders. Common misconceptions include associating bipolar disorder solely with mood swings or viewing it as a character flaw or a choice. It is important to emphasize that bipolar disorder is a medical condition resulting from complex biological, genetic, and environmental factors. By providing accurate information, we can challenge these misconceptions and promote empathy and understanding.

Recognizing Bipolar Disorder as a Medical Condition: Bipolar disorder is a legitimate medical condition that requires proper diagnosis and treatment. It is essential to emphasize that individuals with bipolar disorder are not "crazy" or "unstable." Bipolar disorder is a neurobiological disorder that affects the brain's functioning and can be managed with appropriate medical intervention, therapy, and support.

Highlighting the Spectrum of Symptoms: Bipolar disorder encompasses a spectrum of symptoms beyond mood swings. It includes periods of mania or hypomania characterized by elevated mood, increased energy, and impulsive behavior, as well as depressive episodes marked by sadness, loss of interest, and fatigue. Acknowledging the diversity of symptoms experienced by individuals with bipolar disorder helps dispel the misconception that it is a uniform and easily recognizable condition.

Challenging the "Violent" Stereotype: Contrary to the stereotype that individuals with bipolar disorder are prone to violence, research indicates that they are more likely to be victims of violence rather than perpetrators. It is essential to challenge these unfounded stereotypes and recognize that people with bipolar disorder, like anyone else, have the capacity for empathy, kindness, and non, violence.

Encouraging Open Dialogue: Fostering open dialogue about bipolar disorder is crucial for combating stigma. By encouraging discussions in families, schools, workplaces, and communities, we can break down barriers and create safe spaces for individuals to share their experiences without fear of judgment or discrimination. Open dialogue promotes empathy, reduces stigma, and increases awareness about the realities of living with bipolar disorder.

Promoting Personal Stories: Sharing personal stories of individuals living with bipolar disorder can humanize the condition and challenge stereotypes. Personal narratives provide insight into the daily struggles, triumphs, and resilience of individuals with bipolar disorder. By sharing these stories through various platforms, such as social media, literature, or public speaking engagements, we can foster empathy and understanding among the general public.

Mental Health Literacy: Improving mental health literacy is crucial in challenging stigma and misconceptions. Educating the public about the signs, symptoms, and treatment options for bipolar disorder promotes early detection and intervention. It also equips individuals with the knowledge and skills to support those with bipolar disorder and encourages a compassionate and inclusive society.

Promoting Empathy and Support: Empathy plays a significant role in combatting stigma. By putting ourselves in the shoes of individuals with bipolar disorder, we can better understand their experiences and challenges.

Common stereotypes and myths

Common Stereotypes and Myths: Debunking Misconceptions about Bipolar Disorders

Bipolar disorder is a complex mental health condition that affects millions of individuals worldwide. Unfortunately, it is often surrounded by stereotypes and myths that perpetuate misconceptions and hinder understanding. Dispelling these stereotypes is crucial for fostering empathy, promoting accurate information, and creating a supportive environment for individuals with bipolar disorders. By challenging common stereotypes and debunking myths, we can contribute to a more inclusive and informed society.

Stereotype: Bipolar Disorder is Just Mood Swings

One prevalent stereotype is that bipolar disorder is simply characterized by mood swings. While mood swings are indeed a key component, bipolar disorder is a complex condition that involves distinct episodes of mania or hypomania and depression. These episodes can significantly impact an individual's thoughts, emotions, behaviors, and overall functioning.

Stereotype: Bipolar Disorder is a Character Flaw

Another misconception is that bipolar disorder is a personal weakness or character flaw. In reality, bipolar disorder is a neurobiological condition influenced by a combination of genetic, environmental, and chemical factors. It is not a result of personal shortcomings or moral failings.

Stereotype: Individuals with Bipolar Disorder are Unpredictable and Unreliable

There is a common belief that individuals with bipolar disorder are unpredictable and unreliable. This stereotype ignores the fact that with proper treatment, support, and self, care, individuals with bipolar disorder can lead fulfilling lives and maintain stable relationships. It is important to recognize that stability and reliability can be achieved through adherence to treatment plans and effective coping strategies.

Myth: Bipolar Disorder is Rare

Contrary to the myth that bipolar disorder is rare, it is a relatively common mental health condition, affecting approximately 2% of the global population. Bipolar disorder does not discriminate based on age, gender, or socioeconomic status. It can occur in individuals from all walks of life.

Myth: Bipolar Disorder is Untreatable

Some people mistakenly believe that bipolar disorder is untreatable. In reality, there are various treatment options available that can effectively manage the symptoms and promote stability. These include a combination of medication, therapy (such as cognitive, behavioral therapy or dialectical behavior therapy), self, management strategies, and support from mental health professionals.

Myth: All Individuals with Bipolar Disorder Experience Extreme Mood Swings

Another misconception is that all individuals with bipolar disorder constantly experience extreme mood swings. While some individuals may experience rapid and severe mood shifts, others may have longer periods of stability between episodes. The intensity and frequency of mood swings can vary among individuals with bipolar disorder.

Stereotype: People with Bipolar Disorder are Violent or Dangerous

A harmful stereotype surrounding bipolar disorder is the assumption that individuals with the condition are prone to violence or are dangerous. Research shows that people with bipolar disorder are no more likely to engage in violent behavior than the general population. It is important to separate the symptoms of bipolar disorder from the individual's character, as the vast majority of individuals with bipolar disorder are nonviolent.

Stereotype: Medication Robs Creativity and Personality

There is a misconception that medication used to manage bipolar disorder dampens creativity or alters an individual's personality. In reality, medication is a crucial component of treatment and can help stabilize mood, reduce the frequency and severity of episodes, and improve overall functioning. With the right medication regimen, individuals with bipolar disorder can continue to express their creativity and maintain their unique personalities.

Combating stigma through education and advocacy

Combating Stigma through Education and Advocacy: Empowering Understanding of Bipolar Disorders

Stigma surrounding mental health conditions, including bipolar disorders, often leads to discrimination, misunderstanding, and limited access to support and resources. Overcoming stigma requires a multifaceted approach that includes education and advocacy. By promoting accurate information, challenging stereotypes, and fostering empathy, we can combat stigma, empower individuals with bipolar disorders, and create a more inclusive society.

Education as a Catalyst for Change: Education is a powerful tool in challenging stigma. By providing accurate and evidence, based information about bipolar disorders, we can dispel myths, correct misconceptions, and increase understanding. Educational initiatives can include school programs, community workshops, online resources, and public awareness campaigns. Educating the public about the nature of bipolar disorders, their prevalence, and available treatments fosters empathy, reduces fear, and promotes acceptance.

Challenging Stereotypes: Stereotypes surrounding bipolar disorders contribute to stigma and hinder understanding. Challenging these stereotypes involves highlighting the diversity of experiences within the bipolar community. Emphasizing that individuals with bipolar disorder can lead fulfilling lives, pursue successful careers, and maintain stable relationships counters the negative stereotypes. Media representation plays a crucial role in portraying accurate and nuanced depictions of individuals with bipolar disorder, helping to break down stereotypes and humanize their experiences.

Personal Stories and Lived Experiences: Sharing personal stories of individuals living with bipolar disorder can be a powerful way to combat stigma. Personal narratives humanize the condition, offer insights into the daily challenges faced, and highlight the resilience and strength of those living with bipolar disorders. Hearing firsthand accounts can foster empathy, challenge stereotypes, and reduce the fear and stigma associated with bipolar disorders.

Empowering Self, Advocacy: Empowering individuals with bipolar disorder to advocate for themselves is a crucial aspect of combating stigma. Encouraging self, advocacy involves providing resources and support for individuals to speak openly about their experiences, share their journeys, and advocate for their rights. Through self, advocacy, individuals with bipolar disorder can contribute to public discourse, challenge misconceptions, and promote understanding.

Training for Mental Health Professionals: Mental health professionals play a vital role in combating stigma. Offering specialized training on bipolar disorders equips mental health professionals with the knowledge and skills to provide accurate diagnoses, evidence, based treatments, and compassionate care. Training should emphasize the importance of person, centered care, cultural sensitivity, and addressing the unique challenges faced by individuals with bipolar disorders.

Peer Support and Support Groups: Peer support is a valuable resource for individuals with bipolar disorder. Support groups, both online and in, person, provide a safe space for individuals to connect, share experiences, and offer mutual support. Peer support fosters a sense of belonging, reduces isolation, and helps individuals feel validated and understood.

Peer, led initiatives can also play a significant role in challenging stigma by providing firsthand insights into the lived experiences of individuals with bipolar disorders.

Collaboration with Community Organizations: Collaborating with community organizations, such as mental health advocacy groups, can amplify efforts to combat stigma. Partnering with these organizations helps create a united front against stigma, enables shared resources, and maximizes outreach efforts. By working together, communities can foster supportive environments, promote understanding, and advocate for policies that prioritize mental health support and resources.

School, Based Education Programs: Introducing mental health education programs in schools can significantly contribute to reducing stigma surrounding bipolar disorders. These programs can raise awareness about mental health conditions, provide information on coping strategies, promote empathy, and teach students how to support their peers who may be experiencing bipolar disorders. Education at a young age helps create a generation that is knowledgeable, compassionate, and supportive of mental health concerns.

Personal stories and public awareness campaigns

Personal Stories and Public Awareness Campaigns: Amplifying Understanding of Bipolar Disorders

Personal stories have the power to create meaningful connections, challenge misconceptions, and foster empathy. When it comes to bipolar disorders, sharing personal experiences can play a crucial role in raising public awareness and combating stigma. By combining personal narratives with well, designed public awareness campaigns, we can increase understanding, promote acceptance, and create a more inclusive society for individuals living with bipolar disorders.

The Power of Personal Stories: Personal stories provide a window into the lived experiences of individuals with bipolar disorders. Sharing personal narratives allows individuals to express their challenges, triumphs, and resilience in their own words. Personal stories humanize the condition, challenge stereotypes, and offer unique perspectives that statistics and facts alone cannot convey. Hearing personal stories creates connections, evokes empathy, and reduces the fear and stigma associated with bipolar disorders.

Breaking Down Stereotypes: Stereotypes surrounding bipolar disorders can perpetuate misunderstandings and discrimination. Personal stories break down these stereotypes by presenting diverse experiences and showcasing the full range of human emotions and achievements. Personal stories highlight the complexities of bipolar disorders, showing that individuals are not defined solely by their diagnosis but have multifaceted identities, talents, and aspirations.

Building Empathy and Understanding: Personal stories are powerful tools for building empathy and understanding. By sharing the experiences of individuals with bipolar disorders, we can create a sense of connection and shared humanity. Personal stories allow the public to see beyond the label of bipolar disorder and recognize the commonalities and struggles that individuals face. This increased understanding fosters empathy and compassion, promoting acceptance and support.

Destigmatizing Mental Health: Public awareness campaigns that feature personal stories contribute to destigmatizing mental health, including bipolar disorders. These campaigns challenge the notion that mental health conditions should be hidden or shamed. By publicly sharing personal stories, we normalize conversations about mental health and emphasize that seeking help is a sign of strength, not weakness. Such campaigns encourage individuals to speak openly about their own experiences, reducing the stigma associated with bipolar disorders.

Platforms for Sharing Personal Stories: Various platforms can be utilized to share personal stories and increase public awareness. Online platforms, including personal blogs, social media, and dedicated websites, offer accessible avenues for individuals to share their experiences. Traditional media, such as newspapers, magazines, and television interviews, also provide platforms for amplifying personal stories. Utilizing a combination of these platforms ensures that personal stories reach diverse audiences and maximize their impact.

Collaboration with Advocacy Organizations: Collaborating with mental health advocacy organizations can enhance the reach and impact of personal stories. These organizations have established networks, resources, and platforms dedicated to raising awareness of mental health conditions. By partnering with such organizations, individuals can amplify their personal stories and connect with a wider audience. Advocacy organizations can also provide support, guidance, and resources for individuals who wish to share their experiences.

Coordinated Public Awareness Campaigns: Coordinated public awareness campaigns are essential for maximizing the impact of personal stories. These campaigns utilize various mediums, such as social media, print advertisements, radio, and public events, to share personal narratives, raise awareness, and challenge stigma. Well, designed campaigns incorporate powerful visuals, compelling storytelling, and accurate information about bipolar disorders. They aim to engage the public, generate discussions, and encourage individuals to seek further information and support.

Collaboration with Healthcare Professionals: Collaboration between individuals sharing their personal stories and healthcare professionals enhances the credibility and impact of public awareness campaigns. Healthcare professionals can provide expertise, validate personal experiences, and ensure the accurate portrayal of bipolar disorders. Collaborating with professionals also facilitates the dissemination of accurate information and resources, empowering individuals to seek appropriate help and support.

Living a Balanced Life with Bipolar Disorder

Living a Balanced Life with Bipolar Disorder: Navigating Stability and Well, being

Bipolar disorder is a condition characterized by mood swings, ranging from episodes of elevated energy and euphoria to periods of depression and low mood. Managing bipolar disorder requires a comprehensive approach that focuses on achieving and maintaining stability while promoting overall well, being. By incorporating self, care practices, implementing effective coping strategies, and accessing support systems, individuals with bipolar disorder can lead balanced and fulfilling lives.

Understanding Triggers and Early Warning Signs: Recognizing personal triggers and early warning signs is essential for managing bipolar disorder. Triggers can vary from individual to individual and may include stress, sleep disturbances, medication changes, or substance use. Identifying these triggers empowers individuals to take proactive measures to prevent or minimize the onset of mood episodes.

Developing a Support Network: Building a support network is crucial for maintaining stability and well, being. This network may include healthcare professionals, family members, friends, support groups, or therapists. Having a support system in place provides a source of encouragement, understanding, and assistance during difficult times. It is important to communicate openly with trusted individuals about the challenges and needs associated with bipolar disorder.

Adhering to a Treatment Plan: Following a comprehensive treatment plan is a cornerstone of managing bipolar disorder. This plan typically involves a combination of medication, therapy, and lifestyle modifications. Medications prescribed by healthcare professionals help stabilize mood and prevent mood episodes. Therapy, such as cognitive, behavioral therapy or psychoeducation, equips individuals with coping strategies, stress management techniques, and skills to manage bipolar symptoms effectively.

Consistent Sleep Patterns: Establishing consistent sleep patterns is essential for individuals with bipolar disorder. Disruptions in sleep can trigger mood swings and exacerbate symptoms. Maintaining a regular sleep routine by going to bed and waking up at consistent times promotes stability and supports overall well, being. Creating a calming bedtime routine and ensuring a comfortable sleep environment can aid in achieving quality sleep.

Healthy Lifestyle Choices: Adopting healthy lifestyle choices is beneficial for individuals with bipolar disorder. Regular physical exercise, such as walking, jogging, or yoga, can contribute to mood regulation, stress reduction, and overall mental well, being. A balanced diet rich in whole foods, fruits, vegetables, and lean proteins provides essential nutrients for optimal brain function. Avoiding excessive alcohol or drug use is also important, as substance abuse can worsen bipolar symptoms.

Stress Management Techniques: Managing stress is crucial for individuals with bipolar disorder, as stress can trigger mood episodes. Engaging in stress management techniques, such as deep breathing exercises, mindfulness meditation, journaling, or engaging in hobbies, helps reduce stress levels and promotes emotional well, being. Learning to identify stressors and developing effective coping mechanisms enables individuals to navigate challenging situations more effectively.

Time Management and Routine: Implementing effective time management and establishing routines provide structure and stability. Breaking tasks into manageable segments, prioritizing responsibilities, and setting realistic goals helps individuals avoid feeling overwhelmed. Creating a daily or weekly routine fosters a sense of predictability and reduces uncertainty, which can positively impact mood stability and overall functioning.

Self, Care and Emotional Well, being: Prioritizing self, care is vital for individuals with bipolar disorder. Engaging in activities that bring joy, relaxation, and fulfillment helps maintain emotional well, being. This may include practicing mindfulness, engaging in hobbies, spending time in nature, or connecting with loved ones. Self, care also involves setting boundaries, recognizing personal limits, and learning to say no when necessary.

Communication and Seeking Support: Open and honest communication plays a significant role in managing bipolar disorder. Sharing feelings, concerns, and experiences with trusted individuals, such as healthcare professionals or support networks, helps individuals feel understood and supported.

Wellness strategies: sleep, diet, and exercise

Maintaining wellness is essential for individuals with bipolar disorder. A comprehensive approach to wellness includes incorporating strategies that prioritize sleep, diet, and exercise. These three components play significant roles in stabilizing mood, promoting overall well, being, and managing the symptoms of bipolar disorder. By implementing healthy habits and self, care practices, individuals can enhance stability and improve their quality of life.

The Importance of Sleep: Sleep plays a crucial role in regulating mood and overall mental health. For individuals with bipolar disorder, maintaining a consistent sleep schedule is essential. Disruptions in sleep patterns can trigger mood episodes and worsen symptoms. Aim for 7, 9 hours of quality sleep each night by establishing a regular bedtime routine. Create a sleep, friendly environment that is cool, dark, and free from distractions. Avoid stimulating activities and electronic devices close to bedtime. If sleep disturbances persist, consult with a healthcare professional for guidance and support.

Prioritizing a Balanced Diet: A balanced diet provides the necessary nutrients to support brain function and stabilize mood. Consider the following dietary strategies:

a. Include Nutrient, Rich Foods: Incorporate a variety of whole foods, including fruits, vegetables, whole grains, lean proteins, and healthy fats, into your diet. These foods provide essential vitamins, minerals, and antioxidants that support overall well, being.

b. Limit Processed Foods and Added Sugars: Minimize the consumption of processed foods, sugary snacks, and beverages. These can lead to energy fluctuations, mood swings, and disruptions in blood sugar levels.

c. Omega, 3 Fatty Acids: Omega, 3 fatty acids, found in fatty fish, walnuts, chia seeds, and flaxseeds, have shown potential benefits in managing mood symptoms. Consult with a healthcare professional to determine if omega, 3 supplements are appropriate for you.

d. Stay Hydrated: Drink an adequate amount of water throughout the day to support physical and mental well, being. Dehydration can impact mood and cognitive function.

e. Consider a Balanced Meal Plan: Consulting with a registered dietitian can help develop a personalized meal plan tailored to your specific needs and preferences.

Regular Exercise: Exercise has numerous benefits for individuals with bipolar disorder. It improves overall mood, reduces stress, promotes better sleep, and enhances physical well, being. Consider the following exercise strategies:

a. Engage in Aerobic Activities: Activities such as brisk walking, jogging, swimming, or cycling can elevate mood and boost overall fitness. Aim for at least 150 minutes of moderate aerobic exercise per week or 75 minutes of vigorous exercise.

b. Incorporate Strength Training: Including strength training exercises two to three times a week can improve muscle strength, support bone health, and enhance overall physical fitness. Consult with a fitness professional to develop a safe and appropriate strength training program.

c. Explore Mind, Body Exercises: Practices such as yoga, tai chi, and qigong promote relaxation, reduce stress, and enhance mind, body connection. These exercises can be particularly beneficial in managing bipolar disorder.

d. Find Activities You Enjoy: Engaging in activities you enjoy increases the likelihood of maintaining a consistent exercise routine. Choose activities that align with your interests, whether it's dancing, hiking, playing a sport, or taking fitness classes.

Establishing Healthy Routines: Creating structure and routines in daily life can promote stability and well, being. Consider the following strategies:

a. Set Regular Daily Routines: Establish consistent wake, up and bedtime routines to regulate your body's internal clock. Incorporate activities such as meditation, journaling, or deep breathing exercises to promote relaxation and mental clarity.

Mindfulness and stress reduction techniques

Mindfulness and Stress Reduction Techniques: Cultivating Emotional Balance in Bipolar Disorder

Bipolar disorder is a condition characterized by mood swings and emotional instability. Managing stress and promoting emotional balance are essential for individuals with bipolar disorder. Mindfulness and stress reduction techniques offer valuable tools to enhance emotional well, being, reduce anxiety, and navigate the challenges associated with bipolar disorder. By incorporating these practices into daily life, individuals can cultivate a sense of calmness, improve self, awareness, and enhance overall resilience.

Understanding Mindfulness: Mindfulness involves intentionally bringing one's attention to the present moment, without judgment. It entails observing thoughts, emotions, and bodily sensations with curiosity and acceptance. Mindfulness can be practiced through various techniques, such as meditation, mindful breathing, body scans, or engaging in everyday activities with focused attention.

Benefits of Mindfulness for Bipolar Disorder: Mindfulness has shown promising benefits in managing bipolar disorder symptoms and promoting emotional well, being. Some of the benefits include:

a. Emotional Regulation: Mindfulness helps individuals recognize and regulate emotions more effectively. By cultivating a non, judgmental awareness of emotional states, individuals can respond to challenging emotions with greater clarity and self, compassion.

b. Stress Reduction: Mindfulness practices help reduce stress by increasing awareness of stress triggers and developing healthier responses. Regular practice enhances resilience and reduces the negative impact of stress on mood stability.

c. Improved Self, Awareness: Mindfulness cultivates self, awareness by fostering a deeper understanding of one's thoughts, feelings, and behavioral patterns. This awareness enables individuals to recognize early warning signs of mood changes and implement proactive strategies to maintain stability.

d. Enhancing Cognitive Flexibility: Mindfulness promotes cognitive flexibility, allowing individuals to observe thoughts without getting entangled in them. This shift in perspective can prevent rumination and negative thought patterns often associated with bipolar disorder.

Mindful Breathing: One fundamental mindfulness practice is mindful breathing. It involves directing attention to the breath, observing the sensation of inhalation and exhalation without trying to change it. Mindful breathing can be done at any time, whether during meditation sessions, before important tasks, or in moments of stress or anxiety. It serves as an anchor to the present moment, promoting relaxation and mental clarity.

Body Scan Meditation: Body scan meditation involves systematically directing attention to different parts of the body, observing sensations without judgment. This practice promotes body awareness, releases tension, and encourages a sense of groundedness. Body scan meditations can be guided or self, directed and can be incorporated into daily routines or during times of heightened stress or restlessness.

Loving, Kindness Meditation: Loving, kindness meditation is a practice that involves cultivating feelings of compassion, kindness, and well, wishes towards oneself and others. By offering kind and loving thoughts to oneself and others, individuals with bipolar disorder can cultivate positive emotions, strengthen self, compassion, and enhance social connections. Loving, kindness meditation can be practiced regularly or as needed, and it can contribute to overall emotional well, being.

Mindfulness in Daily Activities: Integrating mindfulness into daily activities is an effective way to promote mindfulness throughout the day. Simple practices include mindful eating, where one focuses on the sensory experience of eating, savoring each bite, and paying attention to hunger and fullness cues. Engaging in mindfulness during routine activities, such as walking, showering, or cleaning, can also enhance present, moment awareness and foster a sense of calm.

Incorporating Mindfulness into Treatment: Mindfulness can be integrated into a comprehensive treatment plan for bipolar disorder. Mental health professionals can incorporate mindfulness, based interventions, such as Mindfulness, Based Cognitive Therapy (MBCT) or Mindfulness, Based Stress Reduction (MBSR), into therapy sessions.

Building resilience and personal growth

Building Resilience and Personal Growth: Nurturing Strength in the Face of Bipolar Disorders

Bipolar disorders present unique challenges that can impact individuals' emotional well, being and overall quality of life. However, it is possible to cultivate resilience and personal growth even in the face of these challenges. Building resilience involves developing coping strategies, fostering support systems, and embracing opportunities for personal growth. By adopting a proactive mindset and implementing effective strategies, individuals with bipolar disorders can navigate the ups and downs of life, enhance their well, being, and cultivate personal growth.

Understanding Resilience: Resilience is the ability to bounce back from adversity and maintain well, being in the face of challenges. It involves adapting to stressors, maintaining a positive outlook, and utilizing effective coping strategies. Building resilience is an ongoing process that can help individuals with bipolar disorders thrive despite the condition's inherent challenges.

Embracing Self, Acceptance: Acceptance of one's condition is a fundamental step towards building resilience. Recognizing that bipolar disorder is a part of one's identity allows individuals to embrace their experiences, acknowledge their strengths, and develop strategies for managing their symptoms. Self, acceptance promotes self, compassion and reduces self, judgment, fostering resilience and personal growth.

Developing Coping Strategies: Coping strategies are essential tools for navigating the challenges associated with bipolar disorders. Effective coping strategies may include:

a. Psychoeducation: Gaining knowledge and understanding about bipolar disorder equips individuals with the information necessary to manage symptoms, make informed decisions, and communicate effectively with healthcare professionals.

b. Self, Care Practices: Engaging in self, care activities that promote physical, emotional, and mental well, being is crucial for building resilience. This may involve prioritizing sleep, maintaining a healthy diet, exercising regularly, engaging in relaxation techniques, and seeking moments of rest and rejuvenation.

c. Stress Reduction Techniques: Adopting stress reduction techniques, such as mindfulness, deep breathing exercises, and journaling, can help individuals manage stress and promote emotional balance.

d. Problem, Solving Skills: Developing problem, solving skills allows individuals to address challenges proactively. Breaking down problems into smaller, manageable steps and seeking support and guidance when needed can contribute to resilience and personal growth.

e. Seeking Support: Building a strong support network is vital for resilience. This network may include family, friends, support groups, or mental health professionals. Connecting with others who have similar experiences can provide a sense of understanding, empathy, and validation.

Fostering Positive Relationships: Nurturing positive relationships is an important aspect of building resilience. Healthy relationships provide emotional support, understanding, and a sense of belonging. Open communication, setting boundaries, and expressing needs and concerns are key elements in cultivating positive relationships.

Seeking Professional Support: Seeking professional support is an essential part of building resilience and managing bipolar disorders. Mental health professionals, such as psychiatrists, therapists, or counselors, can provide guidance, develop personalized treatment plans, and offer support during challenging times. Regular therapy sessions can help individuals explore coping strategies, process emotions, and develop resilience skills.

Embracing a Growth Mindset: Adopting a growth mindset is crucial for personal growth and resilience. Embracing the belief that challenges can be opportunities for learning and growth allows individuals to reframe setbacks as valuable experiences. Cultivating self, reflection and seeking lessons from difficult situations contribute to personal development and resilience.

Setting Realistic Goals: Setting realistic goals helps individuals with bipolar disorders maintain motivation and focus. Breaking larger goals into smaller, achievable steps promotes a sense of accomplishment, builds confidence, and fosters resilience. Regularly reassessing goals and adapting them to changing circumstances ensures continued progress.

Chapter Fifteen

Emerging Research and Future Directions

Emerging Research and Future Directions: Advancing Understanding and Treatment of Bipolar Disorders

Bipolar disorders have long been the subject of scientific inquiry and research, leading to significant advancements in our understanding and treatment of the condition. As research continues to evolve, emerging findings offer hope for improved interventions, enhanced diagnostic methods, and personalized approaches to managing bipolar disorders. This essay explores some of the exciting developments in bipolar disorder research and discusses potential future directions that hold promise for individuals living with this condition.

Genetic and Neurobiological Factors: Recent research has focused on identifying genetic and neurobiological factors associated with bipolar disorders. Advances in genetic studies have uncovered potential genetic markers and variations that may contribute to an individual's vulnerability to the disorder. Additionally, neuroimaging techniques have shed light on structural and functional differences in the brains of individuals with bipolar disorders, providing insights into the underlying neural mechanisms.

Precision Medicine: The field of precision medicine holds promise for tailoring treatment approaches to individual patients based on their unique genetic, environmental, and clinical characteristics. By understanding the genetic variations and neurobiological factors associated with bipolar disorders, researchers are exploring the potential for targeted interventions that can optimize treatment outcomes and minimize side effects.

Early Detection and Intervention: Early detection and intervention are crucial for managing bipolar disorders effectively. Emerging research aims to improve diagnostic methods and identify early warning signs that can help facilitate timely intervention. By identifying prodromal symptoms or markers of risk, healthcare professionals may be able to intervene earlier and potentially prevent or mitigate the onset of full, blown mood episodes.

Predictive Modeling and Digital Health: Advances in digital health technologies and predictive modeling hold promise for monitoring and predicting mood fluctuations in individuals with bipolar disorders. Smartphone apps, wearable devices, and online platforms can collect real, time data on various parameters, such as sleep patterns, physical activity, and mood states. Analyzing these data using machine learning algorithms may enable personalized predictions and interventions, promoting self, management and enhancing treatment outcomes.

Psychosocial Interventions: Psychosocial interventions play a crucial role in managing bipolar disorders, and emerging research is exploring innovative approaches in this domain. Cognitive remediation programs aim to improve cognitive functioning, which can be impaired in bipolar disorder. Social rhythm therapy emphasizes the importance of maintaining regular daily routines to stabilize mood. Integrating psychosocial interventions with pharmacological treatments can enhance overall outcomes and empower individuals to actively participate in their own recovery.

Transcranial Magnetic Stimulation (TMS): Transcranial magnetic stimulation is a non, invasive brain stimulation technique that has shown promise in the treatment of bipolar depression. This procedure involves delivering magnetic pulses to specific regions of the brain, stimulating neural activity and potentially alleviating depressive symptoms. Ongoing research aims to refine TMS protocols and expand its application to different stages and subtypes of bipolar disorders.

Collaborative Care Models: Collaborative care models involve multidisciplinary teams working together to provide comprehensive care for individuals with bipolar disorders. These models integrate mental health professionals, primary care physicians, and other specialists to ensure coordinated and holistic treatment. By addressing both mental health and physical health needs, collaborative care models can improve outcomes and enhance overall well, being.

Long, Term Outcomes and Quality of Life: As individuals with bipolar disorders age, understanding long, term outcomes and factors that influence quality of life becomes increasingly important. Emerging research focuses on factors such as comorbidities, cognitive impairment, social support, and resilience in relation to long, term functioning and quality of life. This knowledge can guide the development of interventions that address specific challenges faced by individuals with bipolar disorders at different stages of their lives.

Intersectionality and Cultural Considerations: Recognizing the intersectionality of bipolar disorders with cultural, social, and environmental factors is an important area of research.

Advances in neuroimaging and genetics

Advances in Neuroimaging and Genetics: Illuminating the Complexities of Bipolar Disorders

Neuroimaging and genetics have revolutionized our understanding of bipolar disorders, shedding light on the intricate interplay between brain structure, function, and genetic factors. Recent advancements in these fields have provided valuable insights into the underlying mechanisms of bipolar disorders, offering hope for improved diagnosis, treatment, and personalized care. This essay explores the exciting developments in neuroimaging and genetics research related to bipolar disorders, highlighting their significance in unraveling the complexities of this condition.

Neuroimaging Techniques: Neuroimaging techniques, such as magnetic resonance imaging (MRI), functional MRI (fMRI), positron emission tomography (PET), and diffusion tensor imaging (DTI), have facilitated the examination of brain structure, connectivity, and activity in individuals with bipolar disorders. These techniques have yielded several notable findings:

a. Structural Alterations: Neuroimaging studies have revealed structural alterations in various brain regions implicated in mood regulation and emotional processing. These include the prefrontal cortex, amygdala, hippocampus, and striatum. Such structural abnormalities may contribute to the disruptions observed in emotional regulation and cognitive functioning in individuals with bipolar disorders.

b. Functional Connectivity: Resting, state fMRI studies have demonstrated altered functional connectivity patterns in individuals with bipolar disorders. Dysregulation within and between brain networks involved in emotional regulation, executive functioning, and reward processing has been observed. These findings provide insights into the neural mechanisms underlying mood dysregulation and cognitive impairments in bipolar disorders.

c. White Matter Integrity: DTI studies have indicated abnormalities in white matter integrity in individuals with bipolar disorders. Disruptions in the connectivity and integrity of white matter tracts, such as the uncinate fasciculus and the corpus callosum, may contribute to the communication deficits observed between brain regions involved in mood regulation and cognitive processes.

Genetic Factors: Genetic research has revealed that bipolar disorders have a strong genetic component. Advances in genome, wide association studies (GWAS) and whole, genome sequencing have identified several genetic variants and risk loci associated with bipolar disorders. Key findings include:

a. Polygenic Nature: Bipolar disorders are considered polygenic, involving the combined effects of multiple genetic variants across the genome. Numerous risk loci have been identified, implicating genes involved in neurotransmitter regulation, calcium signaling, ion channels, and synaptic plasticity. However, the precise role and interactions of these genetic variants require further investigation.

b. Shared Genetic Risk: Genetic studies have revealed shared genetic risk factors between bipolar disorder and other psychiatric conditions, such as schizophrenia and major depressive disorder. This finding supports the notion of a shared biological basis for these disorders and highlights the importance of considering their overlapping genetic influences in research and clinical practice.

c. Rare Genetic Variants: In addition to common genetic variants, rare genetic mutations have been implicated in bipolar disorders. These include rare copy number variations and single gene mutations associated with increased risk. Studying these rare variants provides valuable insights into the specific molecular pathways involved in the development of bipolar disorders.

Gene, Environment Interactions: The interplay between genetic factors and environmental influences is crucial in understanding the complex etiology of bipolar disorders. Research suggests that genetic susceptibility interacts with environmental stressors, such as life events, childhood trauma, or substance abuse, to increase the risk of developing bipolar disorders. Identifying gene, environment interactions can help elucidate the mechanisms by which genetic vulnerabilities are expressed and provide targets for interventions.

Precision Medicine and Personalized Care: The advancements in neuroimaging and genetics research have paved the way for precision medicine approaches in bipolar disorders.

Novel medications and treatment approaches

Novel Medications and Treatment Approaches: Advancing Bipolar Disorder Management

Bipolar disorder is a complex mental health condition that requires a multidimensional approach to treatment. Over the years, significant progress has been made in the development of medications and treatment approaches for bipolar disorder. Researchers and healthcare professionals have been exploring novel strategies to improve symptom management, reduce relapse rates, and enhance overall quality of life for individuals with this condition. This essay highlights some of the exciting advancements in medications and treatment approaches, providing insights into the potential benefits they offer to individuals living with bipolar disorder.

Mood Stabilizers: Mood stabilizers are a cornerstone of bipolar disorder treatment. While lithium has long been a mainstay in managing bipolar disorder, newer mood stabilizers have emerged. For example, anticonvulsant medications such as valproate, lamotrigine, and carbamazepine have shown efficacy in stabilizing mood and preventing relapse. These medications work by modulating neurotransmitter levels and stabilizing neuronal activity in the brain.

Second, Generation Antipsychotics: Second, generation antipsychotics, originally developed for schizophrenia treatment, have also proven effective in managing bipolar disorder. Medications such as quetiapine, aripiprazole, and olanzapine are often used as adjunctive treatments to stabilize mood and manage psychotic symptoms during acute manic or depressive episodes. They work by modulating dopamine and other neurotransmitters in the brain.

Antidepressants: The use of antidepressants in bipolar disorder treatment remains controversial due to concerns about triggering manic or hypomanic episodes. However, in certain cases, under careful monitoring, they can be prescribed cautiously to manage depressive symptoms in bipolar disorder. Selective serotonin reuptake inhibitors (SSRIs) and other newer antidepressants may be used in combination with mood stabilizers to alleviate depressive symptoms.

Psychosocial Interventions: Alongside medications, psychosocial interventions play a crucial role in the management of bipolar disorder. These interventions aim to enhance coping skills, improve adherence to treatment, and promote overall well, being. Some of the widely studied psychosocial interventions for bipolar disorder include:

a. Cognitive, Behavioral Therapy (CBT): CBT focuses on identifying and modifying maladaptive thought patterns and behaviors. It helps individuals recognize triggers, manage stress, and develop coping strategies to prevent relapse and enhance mood stability.

b. Interpersonal and Social Rhythm Therapy (IPSRT): IPSRT combines psychoeducation with the establishment of regular routines and interpersonal problem, solving. It emphasizes the importance of maintaining stable daily routines, including sleep, wake cycles, to support mood stability.

c. Family, Focused Therapy (FFT): FFT involves family members in the treatment process to improve communication, problem, solving, and coping skills. It educates families about bipolar disorder and provides support for both the individual with bipolar disorder and their loved ones.

d. Psychoeducation: Psychoeducation programs provide individuals and their families with information about bipolar disorder, its symptoms, treatment options, and strategies for managing the condition effectively. By increasing knowledge and understanding, psychoeducation empowers individuals to take an active role in their treatment.

Digital Interventions: With the advancements in technology, digital interventions have emerged as a promising avenue for bipolar disorder management. Mobile applications, online platforms, and telemedicine programs provide convenient and accessible tools for self, monitoring, mood tracking, medication adherence, and psychoeducation. These digital interventions can supplement traditional treatments and provide additional support between healthcare visits.

Chronotherapy: Chronotherapy is a relatively novel treatment approach that focuses on regulating the body's biological rhythms to improve mood stability. It involves manipulating sleep, wake cycles, light exposure, and medication timing to reset circadian rhythms.

Early intervention and prevention efforts

Early Intervention and Prevention Efforts: Promoting Well, being and Reducing the Impact of Bipolar Disorders

Early intervention and prevention efforts are crucial in addressing the challenges associated with bipolar disorders. By detecting symptoms early, providing timely interventions, and implementing preventive strategies, the aim is to reduce the impact of the condition and improve overall well, being for individuals at risk or experiencing early signs of bipolar disorders. This essay explores the significance of early intervention and prevention efforts in relation to bipolar disorders, highlighting their potential benefits and providing insights into current approaches.

Recognizing Early Warning Signs: Identifying early warning signs is essential for early intervention in bipolar disorders. These signs may include changes in sleep patterns, mood fluctuations, increased energy levels, changes in appetite or weight, irritability, racing thoughts, or reduced concentration. Increased awareness and education about these early signs can help individuals, their families, and healthcare professionals detect the onset of bipolar symptoms and take appropriate action.

Psychoeducation and Awareness: Psychoeducation programs play a vital role in promoting awareness and understanding of bipolar disorders. These programs provide information about the condition, its symptoms, potential triggers, and available treatment options. By increasing knowledge and awareness among individuals, their families, and the community, psychoeducation programs empower individuals to seek help, recognize early signs, and engage in preventive strategies.

Screening and Assessment: Implementing routine screening and assessment protocols can aid in the early detection of bipolar disorders. Screening tools, such as the Mood Disorder Questionnaire (MDQ) or the Bipolar

Spectrum Diagnostic Scale (BSDS), can assist healthcare professionals in identifying individuals at risk or experiencing subthreshold symptoms. Early detection enables prompt intervention, reducing the risk of progression to a full, blown episode and improving treatment outcomes.

Early Intervention Strategies: Early intervention aims to address bipolar symptoms and prevent the onset of acute episodes. Several strategies have shown promise in this regard:

a. Psychotherapy: Psychotherapeutic interventions, such as cognitive, behavioral therapy (CBT) and family, focused therapy (FFT), can be effective in managing early symptoms and reducing relapse rates. These interventions focus on improving coping skills, stress management, mood regulation, and communication within interpersonal relationships.

b. Medication Management: In some cases, early intervention may involve the judicious use of medications to alleviate symptoms and prevent progression. Mood stabilizers, such as lithium or anticonvulsants, may be prescribed to stabilize mood and prevent manic or depressive episodes. However, careful monitoring and individualized treatment plans are crucial to minimize side effects and optimize outcomes.

c. Supportive Services: Early intervention efforts should encompass comprehensive support services. These may include case management, peer support programs, and access to community resources. These services provide individuals with the necessary support, education, and assistance in navigating the challenges associated with bipolar disorders.

Risk Reduction and Prevention: Prevention efforts aim to reduce the risk of developing bipolar disorders or delay the onset of symptoms. Key strategies include:

a. Lifestyle Modifications: Adopting a healthy lifestyle that incorporates regular exercise, adequate sleep, a balanced diet, and stress management techniques can contribute to overall well, being and potentially reduce the risk of mood disturbances. These lifestyle modifications promote emotional resilience and enhance mental health.

b. Substance Abuse Prevention: Substance abuse can significantly impact the development and course of bipolar disorders. Therefore, prevention efforts should focus on educating individuals about the risks of substance use, promoting healthy coping mechanisms, and providing access to substance abuse prevention programs.

c. Early Intervention in High, Risk Groups: Individuals with a family history of bipolar disorders or a history of subthreshold symptoms are at higher risk of developing the condition. Targeted interventions, such as psychoeducation, psychotherapy, and regular monitoring, can help identify and manage symptoms early in these high, risk individuals.

Chapter Sixteen

Bipolar Disorder and Creativity

Bipolar Disorder and Creativity: Exploring the Complex Relationship

The relationship between bipolar disorder and creativity has long been a topic of fascination and debate. Many notable artists, musicians, writers, and thinkers throughout history have been associated with bipolar disorder, leading to the notion that there might be a link between the condition and creative expression. While there is evidence to suggest a higher prevalence of bipolar disorder among creative individuals, understanding the nature of this relationship is complex and multifaceted. This essay explores the connection between bipolar disorder and creativity, highlighting the factors at play and providing insights into the ongoing discourse surrounding this intriguing topic.

Heightened Emotional States: Bipolar disorder is characterized by extreme mood swings, ranging from manic or hypomanic episodes to depressive episodes. These intense emotional experiences can provide a unique perspective and depth of emotional insight that may fuel the creative process. The heightened emotional states associated with bipolar disorder may contribute to the intensity and emotional resonance found in artistic works.

Enhanced Cognitive Abilities: During manic or hypomanic episodes, individuals with bipolar disorder may experience increased energy, racing thoughts, and heightened creativity. This state of hyperarousal and cognitive stimulation may lead to enhanced problem, solving abilities, increased fluency in generating ideas, and a heightened ability to make novel connections. These cognitive benefits may provide a boost to creative thinking and innovation.

Altered Perception and Sensitivity: Bipolar disorder can influence perception and sensory experiences. Individuals with bipolar disorder may have heightened sensory sensitivity or altered perceptions of the world around them. These altered perceptions can provide a unique lens through which to interpret and represent the world, contributing to the development of innovative and unconventional artistic expressions.

Divergent Thinking and Unconventional Perspectives: Bipolar disorder has been associated with divergent thinking, which refers to the ability to generate multiple solutions or perspectives to a given problem. This cognitive flexibility and willingness to explore unconventional ideas can be advantageous in creative endeavors, allowing individuals to think outside the box and push boundaries in their artistic pursuits.

Catharsis and Self, Expression: Artistic expression can serve as a cathartic outlet for individuals with bipolar disorder, providing a means to channel and express intense emotions. Creative endeavors, such as painting, writing, or music, can offer a safe space to process and communicate complex feelings, contributing to emotional well, being and self, discovery.

Self, Medication and Coping Mechanisms: Some individuals with bipolar disorder may turn to creative activities as a form of self, medication or coping mechanism. Engaging in creative pursuits can provide a sense of purpose, fulfillment, and distraction from distressing symptoms. Creative outlets may serve as a healthy coping strategy, allowing individuals to channel their energy and emotions into productive and meaningful endeavors.

Challenges and Impediments: While there is evidence suggesting a link between bipolar disorder and creativity, it is important to acknowledge the challenges that individuals with the condition may face. Bipolar disorder can be debilitating during depressive episodes, impacting motivation, concentration, and overall functioning. This can hinder creative output and make it difficult to sustain a consistent creative practice. Additionally, the erratic nature of mood swings may lead to inconsistent productivity and difficulties in managing the demands of creative work.

The Role of Treatment: It is crucial to emphasize that not all individuals with bipolar disorder experience heightened creativity, nor is creativity exclusive to those with the condition. Furthermore, it is important to prioritize the well, being and stability of individuals with bipolar disorder over the notion of artistic productivity. Effective treatment, including medication, therapy, and support, plays a vital role in managing bipolar disorder and promoting overall mental health. It is essential for individuals with bipolar disorder to work closely with healthcare professionals to develop a comprehensive treatment plan that prioritizes stability, self, care, and overall well, being.

Historical and contemporary examples

Historical and Contemporary Examples: Notable Figures and Bipolar Disorders

Bipolar disorder, a condition characterized by significant mood swings, has affected individuals throughout history and continues to impact people today. Examining historical and contemporary examples of notable figures who have experienced bipolar disorder sheds light on the complexities of the condition and its potential influence on creativity, productivity, and personal experiences. This essay explores the stories of several individuals, highlighting their achievements and contributions while navigating the challenges associated with bipolar disorders.

Historical Figures:

Vincent van Gogh: One of the most renowned artists in history, Vincent van Gogh is believed to have experienced bipolar disorder. His work, characterized by vivid colors and emotional intensity, reflects the tumultuous inner world he experienced. Van Gogh's artistic brilliance and unique perspectives have left an indelible mark on the art world, even though his struggles with mental health were often misunderstood during his lifetime.

Ludwig van Beethoven: The legendary composer Ludwig van Beethoven is another historical figure believed to have had bipolar disorder. Despite experiencing periods of profound depression and intense mood swings, Beethoven's musical genius thrived. His compositions, known for their emotional depth and intensity, continue to inspire and captivate audiences worldwide.

Virginia Woolf: A pioneer of modernist literature, Virginia Woolf is celebrated for her novels, essays, and experimental writing style. Woolf experienced periods of manic energy and depressive episodes, which significantly influenced her work. Her exploration of the human psyche and internal experiences has left an enduring impact on the literary world.

Contemporary Figures:

Carrie Fisher: Known for her iconic role as Princess Leia in the Star Wars franchise, Carrie Fisher was a prominent advocate for mental health awareness. Fisher openly discussed her struggles with bipolar disorder, using her platform to challenge stigma and promote understanding. Her candidness and humor in addressing her experiences inspired many individuals living with mental health conditions.

Demi Lovato: Pop singer Demi Lovato has been open about her journey with bipolar disorder and substance abuse. Lovato's music and advocacy work reflect her personal struggles, resilience, and commitment to raising awareness about mental health. By sharing her story, she has inspired countless individuals to seek help and support.

Stephen Fry: British actor, comedian, and writer Stephen Fry has been vocal about his experiences with bipolar disorder. Fry's openness and eloquence in discussing his mental health challenges have helped combat stigma and foster understanding. His documentaries and public speaking engagements have educated audiences about bipolar disorder and its impact on individuals' lives.

It is important to note that not all individuals with bipolar disorder achieve fame or recognition. Many people manage the condition quietly, contributing to their communities and pursuing their passions. The experiences of these historical and contemporary figures are representative of the diverse range of talents and achievements within the bipolar community.

While the connection between bipolar disorder and creativity is often romanticized, it is essential to remember that bipolar disorder is a complex condition that affects individuals differently. Not everyone with bipolar disorder will experience heightened creativity or achieve extraordinary success. Furthermore, the challenges associated with the condition, such as mood instability and the need for ongoing management, can impact personal and professional lives.

These examples underscore the importance of understanding bipolar disorder as a multifaceted condition that requires comprehensive treatment and support. They also highlight the resilience and strength demonstrated by individuals living with bipolar disorder, both historically and in the present day.

By sharing their stories, these historical and contemporary figures have contributed to reducing stigma, increasing awareness, and promoting dialogue surrounding bipolar disorder. Their experiences serve as a reminder that individuals with bipolar disorder can lead meaningful and fulfilling lives, pursuing their passions and making valuable contributions to society.

The role of mood states in artistic expression

The Role of Mood States in Artistic Expression: Exploring the Intersection with Bipolar Disorders

Artistic expression has long been associated with the emotional and creative depths of the human experience. The interplay between mood states and artistic output is a subject of fascination and study, particularly in relation to bipolar disorders. Bipolar disorder is characterized by extreme mood swings, ranging from manic or hypomanic episodes to depressive episodes. This essay examines the role of mood states in artistic expression, exploring the ways in which bipolar disorder can influence and shape the creative process.

Manic and Hypomanic Episodes: During manic or hypomanic episodes, individuals with bipolar disorder may experience heightened energy, expansive thinking, and a sense of euphoria. These elevated mood states can fuel creative output, resulting in increased productivity and bursts of inspiration. Artists may experience a surge of ideas, increased motivation, and an intensified drive to create during these periods. The rapid flow of thoughts and enhanced cognitive functioning can lead to innovative and unconventional artistic expressions.

Emotional Intensity and Depth: Bipolar disorder is characterized by intense emotional experiences, and this emotional depth can find expression in artwork. Artists with bipolar disorder may tap into the extreme highs and lows they experience, channeling their intense emotions into their creative endeavors. The range and intensity of emotions can infuse their work with a raw and powerful quality, resonating deeply with audiences.

Transcending Boundaries: Manic or hypomanic episodes may be accompanied by a sense of uninhibited freedom, breaking down barriers and pushing artistic boundaries. Artists may be more willing to take risks, explore unconventional ideas, and challenge established norms. This creative fearlessness can lead to groundbreaking artistic breakthroughs and the creation of unique and thought, provoking works.

Catharsis and Self, Expression: For individuals with bipolar disorder, creating art can serve as a form of catharsis and self, expression. The act of externalizing internal experiences and emotions through artistic mediums can provide relief and release. Art becomes a means of processing and making sense of the intense and sometimes overwhelming emotions associated with bipolar disorder.

Depressive Episodes: While manic and hypomanic episodes are often associated with heightened creativity, depressive episodes can present significant challenges to artistic expression. During depressive episodes, individuals may experience a lack of motivation, decreased energy, and a diminished capacity for creative output. Artists may struggle with self, doubt, decreased interest in their work, and difficulty finding inspiration. The debilitating nature of depression can hinder artistic productivity and impact an artist's ability to engage with their craft.

The Role of Treatment: Effective treatment and management of bipolar disorder can influence the relationship between mood states and artistic expression. Medication and therapy can help stabilize mood, reduce the frequency and severity of mood swings, and enhance overall well, being. By achieving stability, individuals with bipolar disorder may experience a more consistent and sustainable creative practice. It is important to recognize that finding a balance between stability and creative inspiration is unique to each individual and requires ongoing support and collaboration with healthcare professionals.

The Complexities of Artistic Expression: While mood states undoubtedly play a role in artistic expression, it is essential to acknowledge that creativity is multifaceted and influenced by various factors beyond mood alone. Artists draw from their personal experiences, observations, cultural influences, and artistic goals, all of which shape their work. While bipolar disorder may contribute to unique perspectives and emotional depth, it is not a prerequisite for artistic talent or creative expression. Artistic brilliance can be found across a spectrum of mental health experiences.

Harnessing creativity for personal growth

Harnessing Creativity for Personal Growth: Empowering Individuals with Bipolar Disorders

Creativity has the power to transform lives, offering a unique pathway for personal growth and self, discovery. This is especially relevant for individuals with bipolar disorders, who may experience heightened emotional states and possess a deep reservoir of creative potential. This essay explores the ways in which harnessing creativity can contribute to personal growth and well, being for individuals with bipolar disorders, highlighting the benefits and strategies that promote a positive and fulfilling creative journey.

Self, Expression and Emotional Release: Creative outlets provide individuals with bipolar disorder a means of self, expression and emotional release. Through various mediums such as art, music, writing, or dance, individuals can channel their intense emotions, thoughts, and experiences into their creative endeavors. This process allows for catharsis and can foster a sense of emotional balance and inner harmony.

Sense of Purpose and Identity: Engaging in creative pursuits provides individuals with bipolar disorder a sense of purpose and identity beyond their condition. It allows them to define themselves as artists, writers, musicians, or creators, embracing their talents and passions. This sense of identity can be empowering, offering a pathway for personal growth and fulfillment outside of the challenges associated with bipolar disorder.

Coping Mechanism and Stress Reduction: The creative process itself can serve as a coping mechanism, offering a respite from the stressors of daily life and the symptoms of bipolar disorder. Engaging in creative activities enables individuals to focus their energy and attention on something positive, diverting their thoughts away from negative or distressing experiences. The immersive nature of creative work can induce a state of flow, reducing anxiety and promoting a sense of calm.

Enhancing Self, Awareness and Insight: The creative process encourages introspection and self, reflection, leading to increased self, awareness and insight. Through creative expression, individuals with bipolar disorder can explore their own thoughts, emotions, and experiences, gaining a deeper understanding of themselves and their condition. This heightened self, awareness can facilitate personal growth, improved emotional regulation, and better self, management of bipolar symptoms.

Building Resilience and Empowerment: Engaging in creative pursuits can foster resilience and empowerment for individuals with bipolar disorder. The act of creating and sharing one's work requires courage and vulnerability, allowing individuals to confront and overcome fears of judgment or rejection. This resilience carries over into other areas of life, enabling individuals to navigate the challenges associated with bipolar disorder with increased confidence and determination.

Connecting with a Supportive Community: The pursuit of creativity often leads individuals to connect with like, minded individuals who share their passion. This sense of community provides a valuable support network, fostering understanding, empathy, and a sense of belonging. Engaging with a supportive creative community can alleviate feelings of isolation and create opportunities for collaboration, feedback, and shared experiences.

Developing Coping Strategies: The creative process inherently involves problem, solving, adaptability, and resourcefulness. Through their creative journey, individuals with bipolar disorder develop valuable coping strategies that can be applied to other aspects of their lives. The ability to navigate creative challenges, overcome creative blocks, and manage setbacks cultivates resilience and adaptability, equipping individuals with skills that can be utilized in managing their bipolar disorder.

Balancing Structure and Flexibility: Developing a balanced approach to creativity is essential for individuals with bipolar disorder. While the free, flowing nature of creative work may be beneficial during manic or hypomanic episodes, it is important to establish a structure and routine that supports stability and prevents burnout. Setting realistic goals, establishing regular creative practices, and prioritizing self, care can help strike a balance between spontaneity and structure.

Chapter Seventeen

Financial Management and Bipolar Disorder

Financial Management and Bipolar Disorder: Navigating the Path to Stability

Bipolar disorder, a mental health condition characterized by mood swings ranging from manic or hypomanic episodes to depressive episodes, can have a significant impact on an individual's financial well, being. The impulsive behaviors and erratic spending patterns associated with manic episodes, coupled with the challenges of maintaining stable employment during depressive episodes, can lead to financial instability and hardship. This essay explores the importance of financial management for individuals with bipolar disorder, providing insights into effective strategies and resources that can help promote financial stability and well, being.

Understanding the Relationship: Recognizing the complex relationship between bipolar disorder and financial management is crucial. Manic episodes may be accompanied by impulsive and excessive spending, high, risk financial decisions, and poor judgment regarding investments or financial planning. On the other hand, depressive episodes can result in reduced motivation, difficulty maintaining employment, and challenges in meeting financial obligations. Understanding these dynamics enables individuals to proactively address potential issues and implement effective financial management strategies.

Building a Supportive Network: Establishing a support network is vital for individuals with bipolar disorder, especially when it comes to financial management. This network can include trusted family members, friends, or professionals who can provide guidance, accountability, and assistance in making sound financial decisions. Seeking the support of a financial advisor or therapist who specializes in working with individuals with mental health conditions can be particularly valuable.

Creating a Budget: Developing a realistic and comprehensive budget is a key step in managing finances effectively. A budget helps individuals track income, expenses, and savings, providing a clear picture of their financial situation. It enables individuals to identify areas where spending can be reduced or adjusted to meet financial goals. Regularly reviewing and adjusting the budget as circumstances change is crucial for long, term financial stability.

Establishing Financial Goals: Setting financial goals provides individuals with bipolar disorder a sense of direction and purpose. Whether it is building an emergency fund, paying off debt, or saving for a specific purpose, establishing goals helps prioritize financial decisions and motivates individuals to stay on track. Breaking down larger goals into smaller, achievable milestones enhances the sense of progress and accomplishment.

Managing Impulsive Spending: Manic episodes can lead to impulsive spending sprees and financial consequences. Implementing strategies to manage impulsive behaviors is crucial. For instance, individuals can set spending limits, consult a trusted advisor before making significant purchases, or employ a cooling, off period before making impulsive buying decisions. Utilizing cash rather than credit cards can also help limit excessive spending during manic episodes.

Seeking Professional Financial Guidance: Engaging the services of a financial advisor with expertise in working with individuals with bipolar disorder can be invaluable. Such professionals can provide guidance on budgeting, debt management, investment strategies, and long, term financial planning tailored to the unique needs and challenges associated with bipolar disorder. They can offer valuable insights and assist individuals in making informed financial decisions.

Building an Emergency Fund: Creating an emergency fund is an essential component of financial management for individuals with bipolar disorder. Having a reserve of funds set aside for unexpected expenses or periods of financial instability provides a safety net and reduces the stress associated with financial emergencies. Aim to build an emergency fund equivalent to three to six months of living expenses.

Employment Considerations: Maintaining stable employment can be challenging for individuals with bipolar disorder due to the episodic nature of the condition. Open communication with employers, including disclosure of the condition if deemed necessary and appropriate, can help establish a supportive work environment. Exploring flexible work arrangements, reasonable accommodations, or vocational rehabilitation programs can contribute to stable employment and financial security.

Utilizing Financial Assistance Programs: Individuals with bipolar disorder may qualify for various financial assistance programs, depending on their circumstances.

Recognizing and managing impulsive spending

Recognizing and Managing Impulsive Spending: A Key to Financial Stability for Individuals with Bipolar Disorders

Impulsive spending can be a significant challenge for individuals with bipolar disorder, particularly during manic or hypomanic episodes. The impulsive behaviors associated with these mood swings can lead to financial instability and hardship if not effectively managed. This essay explores the importance of recognizing and managing impulsive spending patterns, providing insights into effective strategies that can promote financial stability and well, being for individuals with bipolar disorders.

Understanding Impulsive Spending: Impulsive spending refers to unplanned and often excessive purchases made without careful consideration of long, term financial consequences. During manic or hypomanic episodes, individuals with bipolar disorder may experience a sense of euphoria, heightened energy, and increased impulsivity, leading to impulsive spending behaviors. Recognizing and understanding the triggers and patterns of impulsive spending is a crucial first step in managing this behavior.

Developing Self, Awareness: Cultivating self, awareness is essential for individuals with bipolar disorder to recognize and manage impulsive spending. Becoming familiar with personal spending patterns and understanding the emotional and psychological factors that contribute to impulsive behavior can empower individuals to make more conscious financial decisions. Journaling, self, reflection, or seeking therapy can aid in developing self, awareness.

Implementing Cooling, Off Periods: Introducing a cooling, off period before making impulsive purchases can be an effective strategy. Rather than making immediate buying decisions, individuals can take time to evaluate the necessity and affordability of the purchase. Setting a specific timeframe, such as 24 hours or a few days, allows for a more rational assessment and helps curb impulsive spending tendencies.

Setting Spending Limits: Establishing spending limits is an effective way to prevent impulsive spending. Individuals can set daily, weekly, or monthly spending caps that align with their financial goals and resources. This approach helps maintain a sense of control over finances and prevents excessive spending during manic or hypomanic episodes. Utilizing cash for day, to, day expenses can also serve as a tangible reminder of spending limits.

Creating a Budget: Developing a comprehensive budget is crucial for managing impulsive spending. A budget provides a clear overview of income, expenses, and savings goals, allowing individuals to allocate funds wisely and prioritize financial responsibilities. By tracking expenses and identifying discretionary spending categories, individuals can gain better control over their finances and identify areas where spending can be reduced or adjusted.

Building Supportive Relationships: Surrounding oneself with a supportive network of family, friends, or professionals can play a significant role in managing impulsive spending. Trusted individuals can provide guidance, accountability, and a sounding board for financial decisions. Engaging the support of a financial advisor or therapist who specializes in working with individuals with bipolar disorder can offer valuable insights and strategies for managing impulsive behavior.

Utilizing Cognitive, Behavioral Strategies: Cognitive, behavioral therapy (CBT) techniques can help individuals with bipolar disorder recognize and modify impulsive spending patterns. CBT focuses on identifying irrational thoughts and beliefs that contribute to impulsive behavior and replacing them with healthier, more rational alternatives. Through CBT, individuals can learn to challenge impulsive urges, develop coping strategies, and make informed financial decisions.

Seeking Professional Financial Guidance: Consulting a financial advisor with expertise in working with individuals with bipolar disorder can provide valuable guidance and support. A financial advisor can help create a tailored financial plan, set realistic goals, and provide strategies to manage impulsive spending. They can also assist in developing a long, term financial strategy that considers the unique challenges associated with bipolar disorder.

Strategies for budgeting and financial planning

Strategies for Budgeting and Financial Planning: Navigating the Path to Financial Stability for Individuals with Bipolar Disorders

Budgeting and financial planning are essential tools for individuals with bipolar disorders to achieve and maintain financial stability. The unpredictable nature of the condition, characterized by mood swings and potential financial challenges, emphasizes the need for effective strategies in managing finances. This essay explores strategies that individuals with bipolar disorders can employ to budget effectively and engage in comprehensive financial planning, ensuring a solid foundation for their financial well, being.

Assessing Income and Expenses: The first step in budgeting is to assess income and expenses accurately. Individuals should calculate their total monthly income, considering sources such as employment, disability benefits, or other financial assistance. Concurrently, they should track and categorize expenses, including fixed costs like rent and utilities, variable costs like groceries and transportation, and discretionary spending. This evaluation forms the basis for developing a realistic budget.

Establishing Financial Goals: Setting clear financial goals provides direction and motivation for effective budgeting and financial planning. Goals can include building an emergency fund, paying off debt, saving for retirement, or major expenses like education or homeownership. Clearly defined goals help prioritize financial decisions and allocate resources accordingly, ensuring a focused and purposeful approach to financial management.

Creating a Realistic Budget: Based on the assessment of income and expenses, individuals should create a realistic budget that aligns with their financial goals. The budget should allocate funds to cover essential expenses while leaving room for savings and discretionary spending. It is important to strike a balance between meeting current needs and planning for the future. Regularly reviewing and adjusting the budget as circumstances change is essential for its effectiveness.

Prioritizing Saving: Building savings is a critical aspect of financial planning for individuals with bipolar disorders. Savings provide a safety net during periods of financial instability and help individuals meet unexpected expenses. Aim to save a portion of income each month, even if it is a modest amount. Automatic transfers to a separate savings account can facilitate consistent savings habits and prevent impulsive spending.

Managing Debt: Debt management is an integral part of financial planning. Individuals with bipolar disorders should prioritize paying off high, interest debts and develop a repayment strategy. This may involve consolidating debts, negotiating lower interest rates, or seeking professional assistance to navigate complex debt situations. Avoiding new debt and practicing responsible borrowing habits are key to long, term financial stability.

Tracking and Controlling Spending: Monitoring and controlling spending habits are essential for effective budgeting. Individuals can utilize various methods, such as keeping a spending journal, using budgeting apps, or utilizing online banking tools to track expenses. Regularly reviewing spending patterns helps identify areas where adjustments can be made and promotes conscious decision, making regarding discretionary expenses.

Utilizing Cash Envelopes or Digital Categories: For individuals prone to impulsive spending, using cash envelopes or digital categories can help enforce spending limits. Designate specific envelopes or digital categories for different spending categories, such as groceries, entertainment, or clothing. This technique provides a visual representation of available funds and acts as a reminder to adhere to spending limits. It also encourages individuals to consider their purchases carefully.

Seeking Professional Financial Advice: Engaging the services of a financial advisor can provide valuable guidance tailored to the specific challenges individuals with bipolar disorders may face. A financial advisor can assist in developing a comprehensive financial plan, offer strategies to overcome financial obstacles, and provide expertise in optimizing investment opportunities. Their guidance can help individuals make informed financial decisions and navigate the complexities of financial planning.

Establishing an Emergency Fund: Creating an emergency fund is crucial for individuals with bipolar disorders. Aim to save three to six months' worth of living expenses to provide a safety net during unforeseen circumstances or periods of financial instability.

Dealing with debt and financial recovery

Dealing with Debt and Financial Recovery: Empowering Individuals with Bipolar Disorders

Managing debt and working towards financial recovery can be a daunting task, especially for individuals with bipolar disorders who may have faced financial challenges due to impulsive spending during manic or hypomanic episodes. However, with careful planning, determination, and access to resources, individuals can effectively address their debt and embark on a journey of financial recovery. This essay explores strategies for dealing with debt and achieving financial stability, taking into consideration the unique circumstances and needs of individuals with bipolar disorders.

Facing the Reality of Debt: Acknowledging and accepting the reality of debt is an important first step towards financial recovery. It requires individuals to confront their financial situation honestly, assess the extent of their debts, and understand the impact of interest rates and repayment terms. By facing the reality of debt, individuals can develop a clearer understanding of the path to recovery.

Seeking Professional Guidance: Seeking professional assistance from financial advisors or credit counselors can provide valuable guidance and support in dealing with debt. These professionals can help individuals develop a realistic and manageable repayment plan, negotiate with creditors, and provide strategies to reduce interest rates or consolidate debts. Their expertise can prove instrumental in establishing an effective financial recovery plan.

Creating a Repayment Plan: Developing a repayment plan is crucial for managing debt effectively. Individuals can prioritize their debts based on factors such as interest rates, outstanding balances, or potential legal consequences. They can then allocate available funds towards paying off high, interest debts first, while making minimum payments on other debts. It is important to establish a sustainable repayment schedule and adhere to it consistently.

Exploring Debt Consolidation Options: Debt consolidation can be a useful strategy for individuals with multiple debts. It involves combining debts into a single loan with a lower interest rate or more favorable repayment terms. This simplifies the repayment process by consolidating multiple payments into a single monthly installment. However, individuals should carefully consider the terms and fees associated with debt consolidation options and seek professional advice to determine the best approach for their situation.

Negotiating with Creditors: Communication with creditors is crucial when dealing with debt. Individuals can reach out to creditors to negotiate reduced interest rates, extended repayment terms, or alternative payment arrangements. Many creditors are willing to work with individuals facing financial hardship to find mutually beneficial solutions. It is important to maintain open lines of communication and proactively address any difficulties in meeting repayment obligations.

Developing a Sustainable Budget: A sustainable budget is essential for managing debt and achieving financial recovery. Individuals should closely evaluate their income and expenses to identify areas where spending can be reduced or eliminated. A realistic budget ensures that funds are allocated towards debt repayment while covering essential expenses. Regularly reviewing and adjusting the budget as circumstances change is important to maintain financial stability.

Building an Emergency Fund: Building an emergency fund is a critical component of financial recovery. This fund acts as a safety net during unexpected financial challenges, reducing the reliance on credit cards or loans. Individuals should aim to set aside a portion of their income each month to gradually build an emergency fund. Even small contributions can add up over time and provide a sense of security.

Seeking Employment and Income Stability: Maintaining stable employment and ensuring income stability are essential for addressing debt and achieving financial recovery. Individuals with bipolar disorders may face unique challenges in the workforce due to the episodic nature of their condition. Open communication with employers, exploring flexible work arrangements, or seeking vocational rehabilitation programs can help individuals secure stable employment and create a solid foundation for financial recovery.

Practicing Self, Care and Seeking Support: Self, care is crucial during the journey of debt recovery. Managing debt can be stressful and emotionally challenging, particularly for individuals with bipolar disorders.

Chapter Eighteen

Travel and Bipolar Disorder

Exploring the World: Travel and Bipolar Disorder

Travel is an exciting and enriching experience that allows individuals to discover new cultures, landscapes, and perspectives. For individuals with bipolar disorder, travel can present unique challenges and considerations. However, with careful planning, preparation, and self, awareness, individuals can enjoy fulfilling travel experiences while effectively managing their condition. This essay explores the intersection of travel and bipolar disorder, providing insights into strategies and considerations for individuals seeking to embark on new adventures.

Pre, Travel Preparation: Before embarking on a trip, individuals with bipolar disorder should engage in thorough pre, travel preparation. This includes consulting with healthcare professionals, such as psychiatrists or therapists, to ensure that their mental health is stable and medications are appropriately managed. Healthcare providers can also offer guidance on adjusting medication schedules to accommodate different time zones.

Establishing Stability: Stability is key when considering travel. Individuals should assess their current mental state and determine if it is conducive to undertaking a trip. Stability can be influenced by factors such as recent mood episodes, medication adjustments, or ongoing therapy. Ensuring a period of stability before traveling reduces the risk of disruptive mood swings during the trip.

Researching Destinations: It is essential to conduct thorough research on potential travel destinations. Factors such as climate, accessibility, cultural norms, and availability of mental health services should be considered. Understanding the destination's healthcare infrastructure and accessibility to medications is particularly important to ensure continuity of care during the trip.

Creating a Travel Itinerary: Developing a detailed travel itinerary helps individuals with bipolar disorder maintain structure and stability during their journey. Itinerary planning should include a balance of activities and downtime to avoid overstimulation or exhaustion. Allowing for flexibility in the schedule also accommodates the need to adapt to unexpected changes or mood fluctuations.

Packing Medications and Essentials: Individuals should ensure that they have an adequate supply of medications for the duration of their trip, along with copies of prescriptions and doctor's notes. Medications should be packed in carry, on luggage to prevent loss or theft. It is advisable to bring extra medication in case of delays or unforeseen circumstances. In addition, packing essentials such as a travel, sized first aid kit and a journal for documenting thoughts and emotions can be beneficial.

Practicing Self, Care: Traveling can be physically and emotionally demanding, so practicing self, care is crucial. Individuals should prioritize getting sufficient rest, maintaining a balanced diet, and engaging in regular exercise. Sticking to familiar self, care routines, such as meditation or mindfulness practices, can help manage stress and promote emotional well, being during the trip.

Managing Time Zone Changes: Time zone changes can disrupt sleep patterns and trigger mood fluctuations. To minimize the impact, individuals can gradually adjust their sleep schedule in the days leading up to the trip.

During the journey, maintaining a regular sleep, wake cycle and exposing oneself to natural light can help the body adjust to the new time zone more effectively.

Seeking Support: Traveling with a supportive companion can provide comfort and assistance, particularly during challenging moments. Sharing travel experiences with a trusted friend or family member not only enhances safety but also provides emotional support and understanding. It is crucial to communicate openly about bipolar disorder and discuss specific needs and preferences with travel companions.

Having a Contingency Plan: Despite careful planning, unexpected situations can arise during travel. Having a contingency plan in place helps individuals feel more prepared and empowered. This may include carrying a list of emergency contacts, familiarizing oneself with local healthcare facilities, and considering travel insurance that covers potential medical emergencies or trip interruptions.

Preparing for travel: medication, routine, and support

Traveling can be an exhilarating experience that opens doors to new cultures, adventures, and personal growth. For individuals with bipolar disorders, it is crucial to approach travel with careful planning and consideration. By effectively preparing for travel, including managing medication, maintaining routines, and seeking support, individuals can enhance their travel experiences while effectively managing their condition. This essay explores important strategies and considerations for individuals with bipolar disorders as they prepare for their journeys.

Medication Management: Prior to travel, individuals should focus on effectively managing their medication regimen. It is essential to consult with healthcare professionals, such as psychiatrists or primary care physicians, to ensure medication prescriptions are up to date and sufficient for the duration of the trip. It is advisable to obtain a detailed medication list, including generic and brand names, dosages, and any potential side effects, to carry during the journey.

Carry Medications Safely: Individuals should pack their medications in their carry, on luggage to prevent loss or delays due to checked baggage mishaps. It is recommended to bring an adequate supply of medication, accounting for the trip duration and potential delays. Additionally, carrying medications in their original containers and having a doctor's note or prescription copies can help facilitate security checks and customs procedures.

Adjusting Medication Schedules: Different time zones can disrupt medication schedules. Individuals should consult with healthcare providers to develop a plan for adjusting medication schedules according to the travel destination's time zone. Gradual adjustments to medication timing in the days leading up to the trip can help minimize disruptions and maintain stability.

Establishing Routine: Maintaining a routine while traveling can provide stability and promote overall well, being. Individuals should strive to incorporate familiar routines, such as regular sleep patterns, meal times, and exercise routines, into their travel itinerary. Consistency in routine helps regulate mood and minimize disruptions that could trigger mood swings.

Preparing for Jet Lag: Traveling across time zones can cause jet lag, resulting in fatigue, sleep disturbances, and potential mood changes. To minimize the impact of jet lag, individuals can gradually adjust their sleep schedules a few days before the trip to align with the destination's time zone. During the journey, exposure to natural light, staying hydrated, and avoiding excessive caffeine and alcohol consumption can aid in adapting to the new time zone.

Planning for Mental Health Support: Traveling with a supportive network can enhance the travel experience for individuals with bipolar disorders. Informing trusted family members or friends about the trip, sharing contact information, and discussing the importance of their support can provide reassurance and assistance during challenging moments. Regular check, ins with loved ones can help maintain emotional well, being throughout the journey.

Researching Mental Health Resources: Before embarking on the trip, individuals should research mental health resources available at the travel destination. Familiarizing oneself with local hospitals, clinics, and mental health professionals can provide a sense of security and ensure access to care if needed. Online forums or support groups specific to the travel destination can also serve as valuable resources for connecting with others who have similar experiences.

Packing Self, Care Essentials: It is essential to pack self, care essentials that support mental health and well, being during the journey. This may include items such as a travel, sized journal for expressing thoughts and emotions, relaxation aids like lavender oil or stress balls, comforting items such as a favorite book or music playlist, and any necessary supplies for engaging in mindfulness or meditation practices.

Coping with triggers and mood episodes while away

Coping with Triggers and Mood Episodes while Away: Navigating Bipolar Disorders during Travel

Traveling presents exciting opportunities for exploration and personal growth. However, for individuals with bipolar disorders, it can also bring unique challenges in managing triggers and mood episodes. By employing effective coping strategies and being prepared, individuals can navigate their condition while away and ensure a positive travel experience. This essay explores strategies for coping with triggers and managing mood episodes during travel, offering insights and practical tips for individuals with bipolar disorders.

Identify and Understand Triggers: Recognizing triggers is a crucial step in coping with bipolar disorder while traveling. Triggers can vary for each individual, but common examples include sleep disruptions, stress, changes in routine, and excessive stimulation. Reflect on past experiences and identify triggers that have contributed to mood episodes. Understanding these triggers empowers individuals to take proactive steps to minimize their impact while away.

Plan for Adequate Rest and Sleep: Sleep disruption can disrupt mood stability for individuals with bipolar disorders. While traveling, it is important to prioritize rest and ensure sufficient sleep. This may involve scheduling downtime, creating a sleep, friendly environment in accommodation, and adhering to a regular sleep routine. Packing sleep aids such as earplugs, eye masks, or white noise machines can also help create a conducive sleep environment.

Stick to a Routine: Maintaining a routine, even while away, can provide stability and minimize the risk of mood fluctuations. While travel inevitably disrupts regular routines, individuals can strive to establish a basic structure. This includes consistent wake, up and bedtime routines, meal times, and medication schedules. Having a semblance of routine can help regulate mood and promote stability.

Engage in Self, Care Practices: Prioritizing self, care is essential for managing triggers and maintaining well, being while traveling. Engage in activities that promote relaxation, such as deep breathing exercises, mindfulness meditation, or yoga. Allocate time for activities that bring joy and calm, such as reading, listening to music, or spending time in nature. Being attuned to personal self, care needs helps individuals navigate triggers more effectively.

Establish Boundaries: Setting boundaries is vital for managing stress and avoiding overwhelming situations while away. It is essential to recognize personal limits and communicate them to travel companions. This may involve politely declining certain activities or excursions, ensuring downtime for self, reflection and relaxation, and being assertive about personal needs. Respectful communication and boundary, setting contribute to a more balanced and enjoyable travel experience.

Manage Stimuli and Overstimulation: Traveling often involves exposure to new and stimulating environments. While this can be exciting, it can also trigger mood episodes for individuals with bipolar disorders. It is important to recognize signs of overstimulation and take steps to manage it. This may involve taking regular breaks, seeking quiet spaces for reflection, or engaging in grounding exercises to stay centered and focused.

Utilize Coping Strategies: Develop a repertoire of coping strategies to manage mood episodes while away. These strategies may include deep breathing exercises, journaling, engaging in hobbies, or listening to calming music. Identify coping techniques that have been effective in the past and adapt them to the travel context. Practice self, compassion and patience, recognizing that mood episodes are a part of the condition and can be managed with effective coping mechanisms.

Seek Support: Traveling with a supportive network or seeking support while away can be invaluable for individuals with bipolar disorders. Communicate openly with travel companions about your condition and specific needs. Having someone to talk to, share experiences with, and provide understanding can offer comfort and reassurance. Online support groups or forums specific to bipolar disorders can also serve as sources of support and guidance while traveling.

Balancing adventure and stability

Balancing Adventure and Stability: Navigating Bipolar Disorders with a Sense of Exploration

The desire for adventure and exploration is inherent in the human spirit. For individuals with bipolar disorders, this longing can coexist with the need for stability and self, care. Striking a balance between embracing adventure and maintaining stability is essential for individuals to lead fulfilling lives while effectively managing their condition. This essay explores strategies and considerations for individuals with bipolar disorders as they navigate the delicate balance between adventure and stability, allowing for personal growth and enriching experiences.

Embrace Self, Awareness: Self, awareness is the foundation of balancing adventure and stability. Understanding one's own triggers, limitations, and needs is key to making informed decisions. Reflect on past experiences and identify patterns that contribute to mood episodes. This self, awareness enables individuals to navigate adventure with caution and make choices that support stability.

Establish a Supportive Network: Building a supportive network is crucial for individuals with bipolar disorders seeking to strike a balance between adventure and stability. Surrounding oneself with understanding and compassionate individuals who respect personal boundaries and provide a sense of emotional support fosters a secure environment. Communicate openly with loved ones, friends, or support groups about personal goals, challenges, and aspirations.

Consult with Healthcare Professionals: Collaborating with healthcare professionals is essential in balancing adventure and stability. Regularly consult with psychiatrists, therapists, or counselors to develop a personalized treatment plan that addresses individual needs. Healthcare professionals can offer guidance, monitor medication effectiveness, and provide coping strategies specific to managing bipolar disorders while pursuing adventures.

Develop a Sustainable Routine: Creating a sustainable routine is vital in maintaining stability while embracing adventure. Establish a daily routine that incorporates self, care practices, medication management, and adequate sleep. While routines may be subject to change during adventures, preserving key elements of stability can minimize the risk of triggering mood episodes. Allow for flexibility within the routine to accommodate new experiences and opportunities.

Set Realistic Goals: When embarking on adventures, it is crucial to set realistic goals that align with individual capabilities and needs. Consider the physical and emotional demands of the chosen adventure and assess personal readiness. Setting achievable goals reduces the risk of overwhelming oneself and promotes a sense of accomplishment and satisfaction.

Plan and Prepare: Proper planning and preparation are fundamental in balancing adventure and stability. Research the chosen adventure thoroughly, considering factors such as duration, intensity, and potential challenges. Create a detailed itinerary that includes rest periods, downtime, and self, care activities. Packing essential items such as medications, comfort objects, or grounding tools supports stability and preparedness while venturing into the unknown.

Practice Mindful Decision, Making: Mindful decision, making is crucial when balancing adventure and stability. Before engaging in a new adventure, pause and reflect on how it aligns with personal well, being and goals. Consider the potential risks and benefits, and evaluate whether the adventure is in line with stability and self, care. Mindful decision, making empowers individuals to make choices that support their overall mental health and balance.

Incorporate Self, Care into Adventures: Integrating self, care practices into adventurous experiences helps maintain stability. Engage in activities that promote relaxation, such as deep breathing exercises, journaling, or meditation, during adventures. Take breaks to recharge, connect with nature, or engage in activities that bring joy and peace. Prioritize self, care without guilt, recognizing that it is essential for maintaining stability.

Recognize Limitations: It is important to acknowledge and respect personal limitations when balancing adventure and stability. Understand that certain adventures may be more challenging or triggering than others. Be willing to adjust plans or seek alternative experiences that align with individual comfort levels. Listening to one's intuition and honoring personal boundaries contribute to overall well, being.

Chapter Nineteen

Spirituality and Bipolar Disorder

The Interplay of Spirituality and Bipolar Disorder: Exploring Inner Growth

Bipolar disorder is a complex mental health condition that affects individuals' emotional, cognitive, and behavioral functioning. In the pursuit of holistic well, being, many individuals with bipolar disorder turn to spirituality as a means of finding solace, meaning, and inner strength. This essay delves into the relationship between spirituality and bipolar disorder, highlighting the potential benefits, challenges, and strategies for incorporating spirituality into one's journey of managing the condition.

Understanding Spirituality: Spirituality encompasses a broad spectrum of beliefs, practices, and experiences that connect individuals with something greater than themselves. It is a deeply personal and subjective aspect of human life that can involve religious beliefs, meditation, mindfulness, self, reflection, and a sense of connection to nature or the universe. Spirituality provides a framework for exploring existential questions, seeking meaning, and finding purpose in life.

Finding Meaning and Purpose: Bipolar disorder can be a source of existential turmoil, challenging individuals' sense of self, purpose, and meaning. Engaging in spiritual practices and exploring one's spiritual beliefs can offer a pathway to finding meaning and purpose amidst the ups and downs of the condition. It can provide a sense of hope, resilience, and a deeper understanding of the self and the world.

Cultivating Inner Strength: Spirituality can foster inner strength, resilience, and coping mechanisms that can be beneficial in managing bipolar disorder. Practices such as meditation, prayer, or contemplation can cultivate a sense of calm, grounding, and self, awareness. These practices enable individuals to navigate mood episodes, triggers, and life challenges with greater equanimity and self, compassion.

Seeking Support in Community: Many individuals find solace and support in spiritual communities or religious institutions. These communities can provide a sense of belonging, understanding, and connection with others who share similar beliefs and experiences. Engaging in group activities, attending spiritual gatherings, or participating in rituals and ceremonies can offer a supportive network during difficult times.

Mindfulness and Self, Reflection: Mindfulness practices, rooted in spirituality, can help individuals with bipolar disorder become more attuned to their thoughts, emotions, and sensations. By cultivating present, moment awareness, individuals can observe their mood fluctuations, identify triggers, and respond to them with greater intention and self, care. Mindfulness, based interventions, such as mindfulness, based cognitive therapy, have shown promise in reducing relapse rates and enhancing well, being among individuals with bipolar disorder.

Integrating Spirituality into Treatment: It is essential to integrate spirituality into the overall treatment plan for bipolar disorder. Open communication with healthcare professionals is crucial to ensure that spiritual practices align with evidence, based treatment approaches. Collaboratively exploring how spirituality can complement therapy, medication management, and other interventions can provide a comprehensive and holistic approach to care.

Nurturing a Supportive Mindset: Spirituality can help individuals develop a supportive mindset, emphasizing self, acceptance, compassion, and non, judgment towards oneself and others. This mindset encourages individuals to view bipolar disorder as part of their unique journey, embracing the opportunities for growth, resilience, and transformation that it presents. Adopting a supportive mindset reduces self, stigma, fosters self, care, and promotes a sense of wholeness and well, being.

Engaging in Rituals and Symbolism: Rituals and symbolic practices can play a significant role in spiritual expression and emotional healing. Lighting candles, creating altars, or engaging in specific rituals that hold personal significance can provide a sense of comfort, grounding, and connection to something greater. Symbolism can offer a language for expressing inner experiences and emotions that may be challenging to articulate verbally.

The role of faith and belief in coping with bipolar disorder

The Intersection of Faith and Belief: Nurturing Coping Strategies for Bipolar Disorder

Bipolar disorder is a complex mental health condition that profoundly affects individuals' emotions, thoughts, and behaviors. In the face of its challenges, many individuals with bipolar disorder turn to faith and belief systems as sources of solace, strength, and coping mechanisms. This essay explores the role of faith and belief in coping with bipolar disorder, highlighting the potential benefits, challenges, and strategies for incorporating spiritual practices into the management of the condition.

Understanding Faith and Belief: Faith and belief encompass deeply held convictions, values, and trust in something greater than oneself. They can manifest through religious traditions, personal spirituality, or philosophical systems. Faith provides individuals with a sense of meaning, purpose, and a framework for understanding the world and their place in it. Beliefs shape perceptions, attitudes, and behaviors, offering a lens through which individuals interpret their experiences.

Finding Comfort and Support: Faith and belief systems can offer comfort, solace, and emotional support for individuals with bipolar disorder. The belief in a higher power, divine presence, or universal energy can provide a sense of reassurance and guidance during difficult times. Prayer, meditation, or spiritual rituals can serve as tools for connecting with a higher power and seeking strength and solace amidst the challenges of the condition.

Cultivating Hope and Resilience: Faith and belief foster hope and resilience in individuals with bipolar disorder. The belief in a greater purpose or a divine plan can provide a sense of meaning and a source of motivation during challenging moments. Spiritual teachings often emphasize concepts such as forgiveness, acceptance, and gratitude, which contribute to the development of resilience and the ability to navigate mood episodes with greater equanimity.

Guiding Principles for Self, Care: Faith and belief systems often provide guiding principles and moral values that can inform self, care practices for individuals with bipolar disorder. These principles may include compassion, self, compassion, non, judgment, and kindness towards oneself and others. Integrating these principles into daily life can support emotional well, being, promote healthy relationships, and enhance self, care practices.

Seeking Support in Faith Communities: Faith communities, such as religious congregations or spiritual groups, can offer a supportive network for individuals with bipolar disorder. These communities provide spaces for fellowship, understanding, and empathy. Engaging in group activities, attending religious services, or participating in faith, based support groups can foster a sense of belonging and connection with others who share similar beliefs and experiences.

Coping with Existential Questions: Bipolar disorder can raise existential questions about the nature of suffering, the meaning of life, and the existence of a higher power. Faith and belief systems can provide frameworks for grappling with these profound questions, offering answers, guidance, and philosophical perspectives. Exploring these questions within the context of one's faith or belief system can provide a sense of peace and understanding.

Balancing Faith with Professional Treatment: Integrating faith and belief into the overall treatment plan for bipolar disorder requires open communication and collaboration with healthcare professionals. It is essential to ensure that spiritual practices align with evidence, based treatment approaches. Healthcare professionals can provide guidance on the integration of faith practices with therapy, medication management, and other interventions, promoting a comprehensive and holistic approach to care.

Embracing Personal Agency: Faith and belief systems can empower individuals with bipolar disorder to embrace their personal agency in managing their condition. Belief in one's capacity for growth, transformation, and healing can enhance self, efficacy and promote a proactive approach to self, care. By embracing personal agency, individuals can actively engage in treatment, make informed decisions, and take steps towards well, being.

Mind

,

body practices and their benefits

Unveiling the Power of Mind, Body Practices: Enhancing Well, being in Bipolar Disorders

Mind, body practices have gained significant recognition for their potential to improve overall well, being and promote holistic health. In the realm of bipolar disorders, these practices offer a multifaceted approach to managing the condition and nurturing mental, emotional, and physical well, being. This essay explores various mind, body practices and their benefits in the context of bipolar disorders, shedding light on their potential to enhance self, care, mood stability, and overall quality of life.

Understanding Mind, Body Practices: Mind, body practices encompass a wide range of techniques that engage the connection between the mind and the body. These practices emphasize the integration of mental, emotional, and physical aspects of health, fostering a holistic approach to well, being. Examples of mind, body practices include yoga, meditation, tai chi, qigong, breathing exercises, and mindfulness.

Stress Reduction and Emotional Regulation: Mind, body practices are effective tools for managing stress, a common trigger for mood episodes in bipolar disorders. Engaging in practices such as meditation, deep breathing exercises, or mindfulness cultivates a state of relaxation, reduces anxiety, and enhances emotional regulation. These practices promote self, awareness, enabling individuals to identify early signs of stress and implement coping strategies to maintain balance.

Enhancing Mindfulness and Self, Awareness: Mind, body practices facilitate the development of mindfulness and self, awareness, both of which are valuable in managing bipolar disorders. Mindfulness, based interventions, such as mindfulness, based cognitive therapy, have shown promise in reducing relapse rates and improving overall well, being. By cultivating present, moment awareness, individuals can observe their thoughts, emotions, and bodily sensations, fostering a sense of inner stability and resilience.

Promoting Physical Well, being: Engaging in mind, body practices offers physical benefits that contribute to overall well, being. Practices like yoga, tai chi, and qigong incorporate gentle movements, stretches, and postures that promote flexibility, strength, and balance. Regular physical activity has been linked to improved mood, reduced anxiety, and increased energy levels, all of which are beneficial for individuals with bipolar disorders.

Supporting Sleep Quality: Sleep disturbances are common in bipolar disorders and can significantly impact mood stability. Mind, body practices, such as meditation or relaxation techniques, promote relaxation and facilitate a restful sleep. Implementing a calming bedtime routine that incorporates these practices can improve sleep quality and support overall mental health.

Cultivating Resilience and Coping Mechanisms: Mind, body practices foster resilience and provide individuals with bipolar disorders with valuable coping mechanisms. These practices enhance the ability to adapt to life's challenges, manage mood fluctuations, and maintain emotional balance. Regular engagement in mind, body practices builds a toolkit of effective coping strategies that can be employed during difficult times.

Social Support and Connection: Participating in mind, body practices often involves joining classes or groups, creating opportunities for social support and connection. Engaging with like, minded individuals who share similar goals and challenges can foster a sense of belonging and reduce feelings of isolation. The supportive community aspect of mind, body practices provides a platform for sharing experiences, seeking guidance, and offering encouragement.

Empowering Self, Care: Mind, body practices empower individuals with bipolar disorders to take an active role in their self, care. Engaging in these practices promotes a sense of agency, enabling individuals to prioritize their mental, emotional, and physical well, being. By integrating mind, body practices into their self, care routines, individuals can establish a nurturing and empowering approach to managing their condition.

Accessible and Adaptable: Mind, body practices are accessible to individuals of varying abilities and can be adapted to accommodate different needs. Whether in a group setting, a guided class, or individual practice, these techniques can be tailored to individual preferences and capabilities.

Navigating spiritual crises and growth

Embracing Spiritual Crises and Cultivating Growth: Navigating Bipolar Disorders

Bipolar disorders can often bring about profound spiritual crises, challenging an individual's beliefs, values, and sense of purpose. However, within these crises lie opportunities for profound personal growth and transformation. This essay explores the concept of navigating spiritual crises and the potential for growth in the context of bipolar disorders. It delves into the challenges faced, strategies for managing spiritual crises, and the potential for cultivating resilience and personal development.

Understanding Spiritual Crises: A spiritual crisis is a deeply transformative experience characterized by a questioning of one's beliefs, values, and purpose in life. In the context of bipolar disorders, these crises can be triggered by mood episodes, existential questioning, or the challenges of managing the condition. They may manifest as a loss of faith, a sense of disconnection, or a search for meaning amidst the turmoil.

Acknowledging the Challenges: Navigating spiritual crises within the context of bipolar disorders presents unique challenges. Mood fluctuations and altered perceptions can intensify the impact of crises, making it difficult to find stability and clarity. The unpredictability of bipolar disorders can also undermine one's sense of faith and trust in a higher power or divine plan.

Acceptance and Self, Compassion: Acceptance is a key component of navigating spiritual crises. Recognizing that spiritual crises are a natural part of the human experience, and especially in the context of bipolar disorders, can foster self, compassion and reduce self, judgment. Acceptance allows individuals to embrace their journey and engage in a process of self, discovery and growth.

Seek Support and Guidance: Seeking support and guidance during spiritual crises is crucial. This may involve confiding in trusted friends, family, or spiritual mentors who can provide empathetic listening, understanding, and guidance. Support groups or religious communities may also offer a safe space for individuals to share their experiences, seek comfort, and gain insights from others who have navigated similar challenges.

Cultivate Mindfulness and Self, Reflection: Mindfulness and self, reflection practices are valuable tools for managing spiritual crises. Engaging in mindfulness meditation, journaling, or contemplative practices allows individuals to observe their thoughts, emotions, and beliefs without judgment. These practices foster self, awareness, enabling individuals to explore their experiences, gain clarity, and uncover new insights.

Reevaluating Beliefs and Values: Spiritual crises provide an opportunity to reevaluate and refine one's beliefs and values. Engaging in a process of introspection and questioning can lead to a deeper understanding of oneself and one's place in the world. It may involve examining the congruence between personal beliefs and the challenges posed by bipolar disorders. Reevaluating and modifying beliefs can facilitate personal growth and a renewed sense of purpose.

Embracing Personal Growth: Spiritual crises can serve as catalysts for personal growth and transformation. By embracing the challenges and lessons that arise, individuals can embark on a journey of self, discovery, resilience, building, and expanded consciousness. These crises can deepen self, awareness, empathy, and wisdom, leading to a greater sense of authenticity and wholeness.

Integrating Spirituality into Self, Care: Nurturing one's spiritual well, being is an essential aspect of self, care for individuals with bipolar disorders. Integrating spiritual practices, such as meditation, prayer, or engaging with nature, into daily routines fosters a sense of connection, peace, and inner stability. These practices offer moments of respite, grounding, and spiritual nourishment amidst the fluctuations of bipolar disorders.

Chapter Twenty

Bipolar Disorder and Aging

The Journey of Aging with Bipolar Disorder: Navigating New Challenges and Embracing Well, being

Bipolar disorder is a lifelong mental health condition that affects individuals across their lifespan. As individuals with bipolar disorder age, they face unique challenges and considerations that can impact their well, being. This essay explores the intersection of bipolar disorder and aging, shedding light on the specific challenges, potential adjustments, and strategies for fostering well, being during this stage of life.

The Dynamics of Aging: Aging is a natural and inevitable process that brings physical, cognitive, and emotional changes. For individuals with bipolar disorder, the aging process can interact with the symptoms and management of the condition, requiring careful attention and adaptation.

Managing Medications and Treatment: As individuals age, the management of medications and treatment for bipolar disorder may need to be reviewed and adjusted. Physiological changes associated with aging can affect medication metabolism, necessitating changes in dosages or medication regimens. Regular communication with healthcare professionals is crucial to ensure the effectiveness and safety of treatment.

Recognizing Changes in Symptoms: Aging can influence the manifestation and presentation of bipolar disorder symptoms. Mood episodes may differ in intensity or duration, and new symptoms may emerge. It is important for individuals and their healthcare providers to stay vigilant and monitor any changes in symptoms to ensure appropriate management.

Addressing Cognitive Changes: Cognitive changes, such as memory decline or executive function impairment, can occur as individuals age. These changes can impact the ability to manage the complexities of bipolar disorder. Utilizing cognitive strategies, such as employing memory aids, engaging in cognitive exercises, and seeking cognitive, behavioral therapy, can support cognitive functioning and enhance overall well, being.

Nurturing Physical Health: Maintaining physical health is essential for individuals with bipolar disorder as they age. Engaging in regular exercise, adopting a balanced and nutritious diet, and prioritizing sleep hygiene contribute to overall well, being and can have a positive impact on mood stability. It is important to consult healthcare professionals for personalized recommendations and guidance.

Fostering Social Connections: Social support plays a significant role in the well, being of individuals with bipolar disorder as they age. Cultivating social connections, whether through family, friends, support groups, or community activities, provides emotional support, reduces isolation, and enhances overall quality of life.

Coping with Life Transitions: Aging often involves significant life transitions, such as retirement, loss of loved ones, or changes in living arrangements. These transitions can impact individuals with bipolar disorder and may require additional support and coping strategies. Seeking professional guidance, participating in therapy, and engaging in self, reflection can help navigate these changes with resilience and adaptability.

Incorporating Self, Care Practices: Self, care practices become increasingly important as individuals age with bipolar disorder. This may include engaging in relaxation techniques, pursuing hobbies and interests, practicing mindfulness or meditation, and engaging in activities that promote joy and fulfillment. Self, care practices contribute to overall well, being and serve as tools for managing stress and maintaining mental health.

Accessing Community Resources: Aging with bipolar disorder can be facilitated by accessing community resources tailored to the specific needs of older adults. These resources may include mental health services, support groups, educational programs, and assistance with daily living activities. Utilizing these resources helps individuals navigate the challenges of aging and bipolar disorder while fostering a sense of community and support.

Embracing a Positive Mindset: A positive mindset is essential when aging with bipolar disorder. This involves embracing self, acceptance, focusing on personal strengths, and reframing challenges as opportunities for growth. Cultivating a positive outlook promotes resilience, fosters emotional well, being, and enhances the ability to navigate the complexities of aging and bipolar disorder.

Changes in symptom presentation and treatment needs

The Evolution of Symptom Presentation and Treatment Needs in Bipolar Disorders: Adapting to New Challenges

Bipolar disorder is a complex mental health condition characterized by significant mood fluctuations, ranging from manic highs to depressive lows. While the core symptoms of bipolar disorder remain consistent, the presentation and treatment needs of the condition can evolve over time. This essay explores the changes in symptom presentation and treatment needs in individuals with bipolar disorders, highlighting the importance of adapting treatment approaches to address the unique challenges that arise.

Understanding Symptom Presentation: Bipolar disorder encompasses a spectrum of symptom presentation, with individuals experiencing a range of mood episodes and symptom severity. In some cases, the initial diagnosis may focus on acute manic or depressive episodes. However, over time, the symptom profile may expand to include mixed episodes, rapid cycling, or subsyndromal symptoms. It is crucial for healthcare professionals to consider the evolving nature of symptom presentation to tailor appropriate treatment strategies.

Shifting Mood Episode Patterns: The pattern and frequency of mood episodes can change as individuals with bipolar disorder progress through different stages of the condition. For example, individuals who initially experience infrequent episodes may develop more rapid cycling, characterized by more frequent and shorter, lasting episodes. These shifts in mood episode patterns can significantly impact an individual's quality of life and require adjustments in treatment strategies.

Comorbidities and Symptom Overlap: Bipolar disorder frequently co, occurs with other mental health conditions, such as anxiety disorders, substance use disorders, or attention, deficit/hyperactivity disorder (ADHD). The presence of comorbidities can complicate symptom presentation, as overlapping symptoms may require targeted interventions and integrated treatment approaches.

Cognitive Functioning: Bipolar disorder can affect cognitive functioning, including attention, memory, and executive functions. Changes in cognitive functioning may manifest as difficulties in concentration, decision, making, or problem, solving. Healthcare professionals should consider the impact of cognitive changes when designing treatment plans and implementing cognitive remediation strategies if necessary.

Treatment Resistance: Some individuals with bipolar disorder may experience treatment resistance, where symptoms persist despite adherence to standard treatment approaches. Treatment resistance can be influenced by several factors, including medication side effects, individual variability in treatment response, and the presence of comorbid conditions. In such cases, healthcare professionals may need to explore alternative medication options, augment treatment with additional interventions, or consider specialized treatment programs.

Maintenance and Relapse Prevention: Long, term management of bipolar disorder involves maintenance and relapse prevention strategies. Individuals with bipolar disorder are at higher risk of relapse, particularly during periods of stress, sleep disruption, or medication non, adherence. Treatment plans should include proactive measures such as regular monitoring, psychoeducation, lifestyle modifications, and adherence to medication regimens to minimize the risk of relapse.

Psychosocial Interventions: Alongside medication management, psychosocial interventions play a crucial role in addressing the evolving treatment needs of individuals with bipolar disorder. Psychotherapy approaches, such as cognitive, behavioral therapy (CBT), interpersonal therapy (IPT), or family, focused therapy (FFT), can help individuals develop coping strategies, enhance medication adherence, manage stress, and improve interpersonal relationships.

Tailoring Treatment Approaches: Treatment approaches should be tailored to the specific needs and preferences of individuals with bipolar disorder. Some individuals may benefit from a focus on early intervention and preventive measures, while others may require more intensive interventions during acute episodes. Treatment plans should consider the individual's goals, preferences, and overall functioning, incorporating a collaborative and individualized approach.

Managing comorbid health conditions

Navigating the Intersection: Managing Comorbid Health Conditions in Bipolar Disorders

Bipolar disorder often coexists with other physical and mental health conditions, creating a complex web of challenges for individuals. These comorbidities can complicate the management of bipolar disorder, requiring a comprehensive approach that addresses both the primary condition and the associated health conditions. This essay explores the management of comorbid health conditions in the context of bipolar disorders, highlighting the importance of integrated care, collaboration, and tailored treatment approaches.

Understanding Comorbidities: Comorbid health conditions refer to the simultaneous presence of two or more medical or psychiatric disorders in an individual. In the context of bipolar disorders, common comorbidities include anxiety disorders, substance use disorders, cardiovascular diseases, metabolic disorders, and sleep disorders. The presence of comorbidities can exacerbate symptoms, reduce treatment response, and impact overall well, being.

The Complexity of Dual Diagnosis: The presence of comorbid mental health conditions, such as anxiety disorders or substance use disorders, can complicate the management of bipolar disorder. Dual diagnosis requires an integrated approach that addresses both conditions simultaneously. Integrated treatment programs, such as Dual Diagnosis Anonymous (DDA) or specialized treatment centers, can provide the necessary support and expertise.

Collaborative Care: Managing comorbid health conditions in bipolar disorders necessitates collaboration among healthcare providers from various disciplines. A multidisciplinary team, including psychiatrists, primary care physicians, therapists, and specialists, can collectively address the diverse needs of the individual. Collaboration allows for comprehensive assessment, treatment planning, and ongoing monitoring of both primary and comorbid conditions.

Medication Interactions: When managing comorbidities, it is crucial to consider potential medication interactions. Some medications used for the treatment of bipolar disorder may interact with medications used to manage other health conditions. Close communication between healthcare providers is essential to ensure medication safety, minimize side effects, and optimize treatment outcomes.

Tailoring Treatment Approaches: Treatment plans should be tailored to the individual's specific needs and consider the interplay between bipolar disorder and comorbid health conditions. Flexibility and customization are key, as treatment approaches that work well for one person may not be as effective for another. Integrated treatment models, such as collaborative care, can help address the diverse treatment needs of individuals with comorbidities.

Addressing Shared Risk Factors: Bipolar disorder and certain comorbid health conditions may share common risk factors. For instance, both bipolar disorder and cardiovascular diseases may be influenced by genetic predispositions, lifestyle factors, or chronic stress. Addressing shared risk factors, such as promoting a healthy lifestyle, stress management techniques, and psychoeducation, can positively impact both conditions.

Managing Lifestyle Factors: Lifestyle factors play a significant role in managing comorbid health conditions in bipolar disorder. Adopting a healthy lifestyle, including regular exercise, a balanced diet, adequate sleep, and stress reduction techniques, can contribute to overall well, being and support the management of both bipolar disorder and comorbidities.

Psychoeducation and Self, Management: Psychoeducation is a valuable tool in managing comorbid health conditions. Individuals can benefit from understanding the interrelationships between bipolar disorder and their comorbidities, including how symptoms may interact or exacerbate each other. With appropriate education and self, management strategies, individuals can actively participate in their care, recognize warning signs, and implement coping strategies.

Support Networks and Peer Support: Building strong support networks is crucial when managing comorbid health conditions. This may involve involving family members, friends, or support groups to provide emotional support, share experiences, and offer practical advice.

Support and care for older adults with bipolar disorder

Empowering the Journey: Support and Care for Older Adults with Bipolar Disorder

Bipolar disorder is a lifelong condition that affects individuals across their lifespan, including older adults. The unique challenges faced by older adults with bipolar disorder necessitate specialized support and care. This essay explores the importance of providing comprehensive and tailored support for older adults with bipolar disorder, addressing their specific needs, promoting well, being, and enhancing their quality of life.

Recognizing the Unique Needs of Older Adults: Older adults with bipolar disorder face distinct challenges related to aging, such as physical health concerns, cognitive changes, social isolation, and loss of support networks. It is essential for healthcare providers, caregivers, and family members to recognize these unique needs and ensure that support and care strategies are age, appropriate and responsive.

Comprehensive Assessment: A comprehensive assessment is the foundation for effective support and care. It involves evaluating the individual's physical health, cognitive functioning, medication regimen, social support, and living situation. By understanding the individual's specific circumstances, healthcare professionals can develop tailored care plans that address their needs holistically.

Medication Management: Medication management is crucial for older adults with bipolar disorder. Age, related changes in metabolism and increased vulnerability to medication side effects require careful monitoring and adjustment of medication regimens. Collaborative efforts between healthcare providers, older adults, and caregivers ensure medication adherence, minimize adverse effects, and optimize treatment outcomes.

Psychoeducation and Caregiver Support: Psychoeducation plays a vital role in supporting older adults with bipolar disorder. Providing information about the condition, its symptoms, treatment options, and coping strategies empowers both the individuals and their caregivers. Educating caregivers about bipolar disorder enhances their ability to provide effective support, recognize warning signs, and promote a supportive and understanding environment.

Cognitive Adaptations: Cognitive changes commonly experienced by older adults can impact the management of bipolar disorder. Adjustments may be necessary to accommodate cognitive impairments, such as memory aids, simplifying medication routines, and implementing strategies to support daily functioning. Cognitive adaptations empower older adults to maintain independence and actively participate in their treatment plan.

Social Support and Engagement: Social support plays a significant role in the well, being of older adults with bipolar disorder. Encouraging social engagement through activities, support groups, and community involvement reduces feelings of isolation and provides opportunities for meaningful connections. Nurturing social networks helps to foster emotional well, being and enhance overall quality of life.

Age, Friendly Therapy Approaches: Older adults with bipolar disorder may benefit from therapy approaches tailored to their age and circumstances. Psychosocial interventions, such as cognitive, behavioral therapy (CBT), interpersonal therapy (IPT), or reminiscence therapy, can address the unique challenges faced by older adults and promote emotional resilience, coping skills, and social integration.

Promoting Healthy Lifestyle Habits: Healthy lifestyle habits contribute to the overall well, being of older adults with bipolar disorder. Encouraging regular exercise, maintaining a balanced diet, prioritizing sleep hygiene, and minimizing substance use contribute to physical and mental health. Older adults should receive guidance on healthy lifestyle practices, taking into account their individual abilities and preferences.

Coordinating Care and Collaboration: Coordinating care among different healthcare providers is vital in supporting older adults with bipolar disorder. Establishing effective communication channels ensures that all providers involved in the individual's care are aware of their treatment plan, progress, and any changes in their condition. Collaboration between healthcare providers, caregivers, and individuals fosters a comprehensive and coordinated approach to care.

Chapter Twenty-One

Resources and Further Reading

A Wealth of Knowledge: Resources and Further Reading on Bipolar Disorders

Bipolar disorder is a complex and multifaceted condition that requires ongoing education and understanding. For individuals seeking to expand their knowledge or find additional support, a variety of resources are available. This essay provides an overview of resources and further reading materials related to bipolar disorders, offering a starting point for individuals interested in deepening their understanding and accessing valuable information.

National Alliance on Mental Illness (NAMI): NAMI is a renowned organization dedicated to supporting individuals and families affected by mental health conditions, including bipolar disorder. Their website offers a wealth of information, including educational resources, support groups, helpline services, and advocacy opportunities. NAMI provides a comprehensive understanding of bipolar disorder, treatment options, and strategies for managing the condition.

International Bipolar Foundation (IBPF): IBPF is an organization committed to improving the lives of those living with bipolar disorder through education, support, and research. Their website offers informative articles, webinars, and resources addressing various aspects of bipolar disorder. Additionally, IBPF hosts online support communities, allowing individuals to connect with peers and share their experiences.

Books on Bipolar Disorder: Several books provide in, depth knowledge and personal perspectives on bipolar disorder. "An Unquiet Mind" by Kay Redfield Jamison offers a memoir of her own experiences as a clinical psychologist living with bipolar disorder. "The Bipolar Disorder Survival Guide" by David J. Miklowitz provides practical advice and strategies for managing bipolar disorder effectively. These books offer insights into the condition and serve as empowering resources for individuals and their loved ones.

Scientific Literature: Academic journals and research papers offer evidence, based information on bipolar disorder. Peer, reviewed journals such as the Journal of Affective Disorders, Bipolar Disorders, and the Journal of Clinical Psychiatry publish studies on various aspects of bipolar disorder, including treatment approaches, symptom management, and neurobiological findings. Accessing scientific literature provides individuals with the most up, to, date research and insights into the condition.

Online Forums and Support Groups: Online forums and support groups provide platforms for individuals with bipolar disorder to connect, share experiences, and seek support. Websites such as Psych Central and Bipolar World offer discussion boards where individuals can engage in conversations, ask questions, and find comfort in knowing they are not alone. However, it is essential to approach online forums with caution and verify information with reliable sources.

Mental Health Websites: Several reputable websites offer comprehensive information on bipolar disorder, its symptoms, treatment options, and management strategies. Websites such as Mayo Clinic, WebMD, and MedlinePlus provide user, friendly resources that cover various aspects of bipolar disorder, including its causes, diagnostic criteria, and available treatments. These websites serve as valuable references for individuals seeking reliable information.

Government Health Agencies: Government health agencies, such as the National Institute of Mental Health (NIMH) and the Centers for Disease Control and Prevention (CDC), offer authoritative information on bipolar disorder. These agencies provide resources, fact sheets, and research updates, ensuring individuals have access to the latest information on the condition and its management.

Mental Health Apps: With the increasing popularity of smartphones, mental health apps have become readily accessible tools for individuals with bipolar disorder. Apps like eMoods, Moodpath, and Daylio help users track their moods, identify triggers, and monitor medication adherence. These apps offer a convenient way to monitor one's well, being and provide insights into patterns and trends.

Educational materials for patients, families, and professionals

Education plays a vital role in raising awareness, understanding, and providing support for individuals living with bipolar disorder. It also helps families and healthcare professionals navigate the complexities of this condition. Below we will explore various educational materials available for patients, families, and professionals that provide valuable insights into bipolar disorder. These resources aim to empower individuals by offering accurate information, practical guidance, and a sense of community.

Books:

Books are valuable resources for gaining in, depth knowledge about bipolar disorder. Several renowned authors have shared their expertise and personal experiences to shed light on the condition. For patients, books like "An Unquiet Mind" by Kay Redfield Jamison and "Madness: A Bipolar Life" by Marya Hornbacher offer personal narratives that inspire hope and resilience. For families and professionals, "The Bipolar Disorder Survival Guide" by David J. Miklowitz and "Bipolar II Disorder Workbook" by Stephanie McMurrich Roberts provide practical strategies for managing symptoms and supporting loved ones.

Websites and Online Platforms:

The internet has become a treasure trove of information and support for individuals affected by bipolar disorder. Websites like the National Alliance on Mental Illness (NAMI) and the Depression and Bipolar Support Alliance (DBSA) offer extensive resources, including fact sheets, articles, and online communities. These platforms facilitate peer support, share personal stories, and provide practical advice on various aspects of living with bipolar disorder.

Online Courses and Webinars:

Online courses and webinars provide structured learning opportunities for patients, families, and professionals. Organizations like the International Bipolar Foundation and PsychHub offer free or low, cost courses covering topics such as symptom management, medication adherence, and strategies for building resilience. These courses are designed to enhance understanding, promote self, care, and empower individuals with the necessary knowledge and skills to navigate the challenges associated with bipolar disorder.

Support Groups and Peer Networks:

Support groups and peer networks create a sense of community for individuals living with bipolar disorder. Organizations like DBSA and NAMI facilitate local support groups where individuals can connect, share experiences, and learn from one another. These groups provide a safe space for discussing challenges, receiving support, and accessing valuable resources.

Online forums and social media groups also offer virtual support networks, connecting individuals from diverse backgrounds and geographical locations.

Professional Training and Continuing Education:

Bipolar disorder requires competent professionals who can provide accurate diagnoses, effective treatment, and ongoing support. Various organizations offer professional training and continuing education programs to enhance the knowledge and skills of healthcare providers. These programs cover topics such as evidence, based treatments, cultural competency, and the latest research in bipolar disorder. The International Society for Bipolar Disorders (ISBD) and the American Psychiatric Association (APA) are prominent organizations offering educational opportunities for mental health professionals.

Research Journals and Publications:

Academic journals and research publications are crucial for staying updated on the latest advancements in the field of bipolar disorder. Journals like "Bipolar Disorders" and "Journal of Affective Disorders" publish peer, reviewed research articles that contribute to the scientific understanding of the condition. These publications provide insights into emerging treatments, diagnostic tools, and the underlying neurobiological mechanisms, informing professionals and researchers alike.

Advocacy and support opportunities

Empowering Change: Advocacy and Support Opportunities for Bipolar Disorders

Advocacy and support play a crucial role in raising awareness, promoting understanding, and improving the lives of individuals living with bipolar disorder. Below we will explore the various advocacy and support opportunities available for individuals, families, and communities affected by bipolar disorders. These initiatives aim to drive change, reduce stigma, and ensure access to quality care and resources.

Nonprofit Organizations:

Nonprofit organizations are at the forefront of advocacy and support efforts for bipolar disorders. The National Alliance on Mental Illness (NAMI) and the Depression and Bipolar Support Alliance (DBSA) are prominent organizations that provide a range of resources, educational programs, and support networks. They also advocate for policy changes, promote research funding, and raise public awareness about bipolar disorders.

Mental Health Advocacy:

Advocacy involves speaking up and taking action to improve the lives of individuals affected by bipolar disorder. Mental health advocates work to promote understanding, fight stigma, and push for better access to treatment and support services. These advocates engage in activities such as lobbying for policy changes, organizing awareness campaigns, and sharing personal stories to increase public understanding.

Peer Support Programs:

Peer support programs offer a unique form of support by connecting individuals who have firsthand experience with bipolar disorder. Programs like the DBSA's "Peer Specialist Training" and the Wellness Recovery Action Plan (WRAP) provide training for individuals to become peer supporters. Peer support offers empathy, understanding, and practical guidance from those who have walked a similar path, fostering a sense of community and empowerment.

Online Communities:

The internet has revolutionized the way people connect and access support. Online communities dedicated to bipolar disorders provide a platform for individuals to share experiences, seek advice, and offer support to one another. Websites, forums, and social media groups like Reddit's r/bipolar and Psych Central's Bipolar Support Community facilitate online discussions, resource sharing, and virtual support networks.

Public Awareness Campaigns:

Public awareness campaigns aim to challenge stereotypes, educate the public, and reduce stigma surrounding bipolar disorders. These campaigns often feature personal stories, educational materials, and engaging social media content to reach a wide audience. Initiatives such as "Bipolar Awareness Month" and "Mental Health Awareness Week" provide opportunities to engage in conversations, dispel myths, and promote understanding.

Policy and Legislative Advocacy:

Advocacy efforts extend to the policy and legislative level to improve the lives of individuals with bipolar disorder. Advocacy organizations work to shape mental health policies, increase funding for research and treatment, and promote legislation that ensures access to necessary healthcare services. These efforts focus on advocating for mental health parity, improved insurance coverage, and increased availability of community, based support programs.

Research Participation:

Research participation provides an opportunity for individuals with bipolar disorder to contribute to scientific advancements and treatment options. Clinical trials and research studies rely on the participation of individuals with bipolar disorder to gather data and test new interventions.

Participating in research not only benefits the individual but also contributes to the collective knowledge and understanding of the condition.

Workforce Support and Accommodations:

Advocacy initiatives also aim to create supportive environments in the workplace. Employers and employees can work together to provide accommodations, such as flexible schedules, modified work environments, and mental health resources, to support individuals with bipolar disorder in their professional endeavors. Organizations like the Job Accommodation Network (JAN) offer resources and guidance for employers and employees navigating these accommodations.

Chapter Twenty-Two

Bipolar Disorder and the Legal System

Bipolar disorder is a complex mental health condition that can have significant implications for individuals within the legal system. This essay explores the intersection between bipolar disorder and the legal system, highlighting the challenges individuals with bipolar disorder may face and the potential support and accommodations available to them. It is essential to ensure fairness, access to justice, and appropriate treatment for individuals with bipolar disorder who come into contact with the legal system.

Understanding Bipolar Disorder:

Bipolar disorder is characterized by extreme mood swings, including manic episodes (elevated mood, increased energy) and depressive episodes (profound sadness, lack of energy). These mood swings can impact cognitive functioning, decision, making, and behavior. It is important for legal professionals to have a basic understanding of bipolar disorder to ensure fair treatment and appropriate support.

Competence to Stand Trial:

One legal consideration is the competence of individuals with bipolar disorder to stand trial. Competence refers to the ability to understand the nature of the legal proceedings and assist in one's defense. In some cases, bipolar symptoms may impair an individual's ability to fully comprehend the charges and participate in their defense. In such situations, a competency evaluation may be necessary to determine if the individual can stand trial or requires treatment and stabilization first.

Mental Health Diversion Programs:

To address the specific needs of individuals with bipolar disorder who come into contact with the legal system, some jurisdictions have established mental health diversion programs. These programs aim to provide treatment and support instead of traditional criminal penalties. By diverting individuals to mental health services, such as counseling, medication management, and rehabilitation programs, these initiatives seek to address the underlying mental health issues that may contribute to criminal behavior.

Courtroom Accommodations:

Individuals with bipolar disorder may require accommodations in the courtroom to ensure a fair trial. For example, adjustments to scheduling, breaks during proceedings, or modifications to the physical environment can help minimize stress and promote the individual's ability to participate effectively. These accommodations align with the principle of equal access to justice for all individuals, regardless of their mental health status.

Sentencing Considerations:

In cases where individuals with bipolar disorder are convicted, it is crucial for judges and legal professionals to consider the impact of the disorder on sentencing decisions. Bipolar disorder's episodic nature and the potential for mood fluctuations may necessitate tailored approaches to sentencing, such as alternative sentencing options, mental health treatment programs, or probation with mental health monitoring. This approach recognizes the importance of addressing the underlying mental health condition while holding individuals accountable for their actions.

Treatment in Correctional Facilities:

For individuals with bipolar disorder who are incarcerated, access to adequate mental health treatment is vital. Correctional facilities should have protocols in place to identify individuals with bipolar disorder, provide necessary medications, and offer therapeutic interventions to manage symptoms and promote stability. Collaboration between mental health professionals and correctional staff is essential to ensure appropriate care within the confines of the correctional system.

Community Reintegration:

Upon release from incarceration, individuals with bipolar disorder face unique challenges in reintegrating into society. Transitional support programs that provide access to mental health services, housing assistance, vocational training, and community support networks can enhance successful reintegration. These programs address the broader social and psychological factors that contribute to the individual's overall well, being and reduce the likelihood of recidivism.

Education and Training for Legal Professionals:

Enhancing education and training for legal professionals on bipolar disorder can foster greater understanding and empathy when interacting with individuals with bipolar disorder. Continuing education programs, workshops, and resources that provide insights into the challenges faced by individuals with bipolar disorder can improve the overall fairness and sensitivity within the legal system.

Mental health law and involuntary treatment

Balancing Autonomy and Care: Mental Health Law and Involuntary Treatment for Bipolar Disorders

Mental health law plays a critical role in protecting the rights and well, being of individuals with bipolar disorder. In some cases, involuntary treatment may be necessary to ensure the safety and stability of individuals experiencing severe symptoms. This essay explores the complex intersection of mental health law and involuntary treatment in relation to bipolar disorders. It examines the legal framework, ethical considerations, and challenges involved in balancing the autonomy of individuals with the duty to provide necessary care.

Legal Framework:

Mental health laws vary across jurisdictions but generally provide a legal framework for the involuntary treatment of individuals with mental health conditions, including bipolar disorder. These laws outline the criteria for involuntary hospitalization, assessment procedures, and the duration of treatment. They aim to strike a balance between protecting the individual's rights and safeguarding public safety.

Criteria for Involuntary Treatment:

The criteria for involuntary treatment typically require evidence that the individual poses a risk of harm to themselves or others due to their mental health condition. The specific criteria may vary, but common elements include the presence of severe symptoms, impaired judgment, and a lack of insight into the need for treatment. These criteria serve as safeguards to ensure that involuntary treatment is justified and necessary.

Role of Mental Health Professionals:

Mental health professionals, including psychiatrists and psychologists, play a crucial role in assessing individuals for involuntary treatment. They evaluate the severity of symptoms, the risk of harm, and the individual's capacity to make informed decisions regarding their treatment. Their expertise and professional judgment are essential in determining whether involuntary treatment is justified and in providing appropriate care.

Ethical Considerations:

Involuntary treatment raises ethical considerations regarding individual autonomy, dignity, and the right to make decisions about one's own healthcare. Balancing the need for treatment with respect for an individual's rights can be challenging. Mental health professionals must ensure that the decision to initiate involuntary treatment is made with the utmost care and consideration, adhering to ethical principles such as beneficence, respect for autonomy, and least restrictive intervention.

Safeguards and Procedural Protections:

To protect the rights of individuals undergoing involuntary treatment, mental health laws often include safeguards and procedural protections. These may include regular reviews of treatment, the involvement of independent review boards, and the provision of legal representation. These safeguards help ensure that the decision for involuntary treatment is continually evaluated and that the individual's rights are respected throughout the treatment process.

Alternatives to Involuntary Treatment:

Efforts are being made to explore alternative approaches to involuntary treatment for individuals with bipolar disorder. Collaborative care models, crisis intervention teams, and intensive community, based services aim to provide early intervention, support, and resources to individuals experiencing acute symptoms. These approaches focus on preventing crises, enhancing access to voluntary treatment, and promoting community integration.

Advocacy and Legal Rights:

Individuals with bipolar disorder have the right to advocate for their own care, voice their treatment preferences, and participate in decisions regarding their treatment. Laws and legal frameworks should support these rights, ensuring that individuals are provided with information, supported in decision, making processes, and given the opportunity to express their concerns and preferences regarding treatment options.

Ongoing Challenges:

Involuntary treatment for bipolar disorder presents ongoing challenges. Striking the right balance between individual autonomy and ensuring necessary care remains a complex task. The availability of resources, access to appropriate treatment facilities, and the need for ongoing monitoring and support are areas that require continuous attention and improvement within mental health systems.

Navigating the criminal justice system

Navigating the criminal justice system can be a complex and challenging experience for individuals with bipolar disorder. Bipolar disorder is a mental health condition characterized by severe mood swings, including manic and depressive episodes. This essay explores the unique challenges faced by individuals with bipolar disorder within the criminal justice system and highlights the importance of understanding and accommodating their specific needs.

Recognizing the Impact of Bipolar Disorder:

It is crucial for legal professionals to recognize the impact of bipolar disorder on individuals' behavior and decision, making processes. Bipolar disorder can significantly affect an individual's judgment, impulsivity, and ability to control emotions, potentially leading to behaviors that may be viewed as criminal. Understanding the underlying mental health condition is essential in order to respond appropriately and address the root causes of certain behaviors.

Mental Health Screening and Diversion Programs:

Early identification of bipolar disorder within the criminal justice system is crucial for appropriate intervention. Mental health screening tools can be implemented during the initial stages of arrest or during the pre, trial process to identify individuals with potential mental health conditions, including bipolar disorder. Diversion programs that focus on mental health treatment and support, rather than punitive measures, can provide an alternative approach for individuals with bipolar disorder involved in non, violent offenses.

Competence to Stand Trial:

Assessing an individual's competence to stand trial is an important consideration in cases involving bipolar disorder. Competence refers to an individual's ability to understand the charges against them and effectively participate in their own defense. If the individual's bipolar symptoms significantly impair their cognitive functioning, a competency evaluation may be necessary to determine their ability to comprehend and actively engage in the legal proceedings.

Courtroom Accommodations:

Individuals with bipolar disorder may require courtroom accommodations to ensure their fair participation in legal proceedings. Accommodations can include flexible scheduling to manage medication regimens or minimize fatigue, breaks during proceedings to address anxiety or mood instability, or adjustments to the physical environment to reduce sensory triggers. These accommodations help ensure that individuals can effectively communicate and comprehend the legal process.

Mental Health Treatment in Correctional Facilities:

When individuals with bipolar disorder are incarcerated, it is crucial to provide appropriate mental health treatment and support. Correctional facilities should have mental health professionals who can assess and manage bipolar symptoms, prescribe necessary medications, and provide therapeutic interventions. Collaborating with mental health experts can help ensure continuity of care, promote stability, and reduce the risk of exacerbating symptoms during incarceration.

Community Reintegration and Support:

Upon release from incarceration, individuals with bipolar disorder face challenges in reintegrating into society. Community support programs, including mental health services, housing assistance, vocational training, and peer support networks, can facilitate successful reintegration. These programs aim to address the broader social and psychological factors that contribute to individuals' overall well, being and reduce the likelihood of recidivism.

Sensitivity and Training for Legal Professionals:

Training legal professionals in understanding bipolar disorder and related mental health conditions is crucial for fair and equitable treatment within the criminal justice system. Enhancing their knowledge about the symptoms, challenges, and available support resources can lead to more compassionate and effective interactions with individuals with bipolar disorder. This training can help reduce stigma, facilitate better communication, and support appropriate decision, making within the legal process.

Collaboration between Mental Health and Legal Systems:

Collaboration between the mental health and legal systems is essential to ensure comprehensive care and support for individuals with bipolar disorder involved in the criminal justice system. Regular communication and cooperation between mental health professionals, probation officers, parole officers, and legal professionals can help coordinate appropriate treatment plans, monitor medication compliance, and facilitate successful reintegration.

Legal rights and resources for individuals with bipolar disorder

Individuals with bipolar disorder face unique challenges within the legal system, but they also possess legal rights and access to resources to ensure fair treatment and support. This essay explores the legal rights and resources available for individuals with bipolar disorder, emphasizing their empowerment, advocacy, and access to justice.

Right to Equality:

Individuals with bipolar disorder are entitled to equal treatment under the law. This means they should not face discrimination or prejudice solely based on their mental health condition. Legal protections, such as the Americans with Disabilities Act (ADA) in the United States, aim to ensure equal opportunities and access to employment, education, housing, and public services for individuals with bipolar disorder.

Right to Privacy and Confidentiality:

Individuals with bipolar disorder have a right to privacy and confidentiality regarding their medical information. Legal frameworks, such as the Health Insurance Portability and Accountability Act (HIPAA) in the United States, safeguard their health records from unauthorized disclosure. This protection enables individuals to seek appropriate treatment without fear of stigma or discrimination.

Informed Consent and Medical Decision, Making:

Individuals with bipolar disorder have the right to be informed and actively participate in their medical decisions. Healthcare providers should provide clear information about treatment options, risks, benefits, and alternatives. Informed consent ensures that individuals with bipolar disorder can make autonomous decisions regarding their mental health care, including medication choices, therapy, and treatment plans.

Disability Accommodations:

Bipolar disorder can impact an individual's daily functioning and work capacity. Disability laws, such as the Rehabilitation Act and the ADA, require employers, educational institutions, and public entities to provide reasonable accommodations to individuals with bipolar disorder. Accommodations may include flexible work schedules, modified job duties, additional breaks, or adjustments in academic settings to support individuals in fulfilling their responsibilities.

Legal Aid and Advocacy Organizations:

Legal aid and advocacy organizations play a vital role in supporting individuals with bipolar disorder. These organizations provide legal assistance, guidance, and advocacy for individuals who may face legal challenges related to their mental health condition. They offer resources, information, and representation to ensure that individuals with bipolar disorder understand their rights and can access justice.

Crisis Intervention and Mental Health Courts:

In some jurisdictions, specialized crisis intervention teams and mental health courts have been established to address the unique needs of individuals with mental health conditions, including bipolar disorder. Crisis intervention teams consist of trained professionals who respond to mental health crises and aim to divert individuals from unnecessary arrests or incarceration. Mental health courts focus on treatment and support, offering alternatives to traditional criminal proceedings.

Advance Directives and Mental Health Treatment:

Advance directives allow individuals to outline their preferences for mental health treatment in advance, ensuring their wishes are respected even during periods of incapacitation or crisis. These directives can include specific instructions regarding hospitalization, medication preferences, and treatment preferences. Advance directives empower individuals with bipolar disorder to maintain a level of control over their treatment decisions.

Self, Advocacy and Support Networks:

Self, advocacy is a crucial aspect of navigating the legal system for individuals with bipolar disorder. Joining support networks, such as local support groups or online communities, allows individuals to connect with others facing similar challenges, share experiences, and exchange information. These networks can provide emotional support, practical guidance, and empowerment in asserting legal rights.

Chapter Twenty-Three

Bipolar Disorder and Sleep

The Intricate Relationship Between Bipolar Disorder and Sleep

Sleep plays a critical role in our overall well, being, and its impact on mental health cannot be overstated. For individuals with bipolar disorder, sleep disturbances can have profound effects on mood regulation and symptom management. This essay explores the intricate relationship between bipolar disorder and sleep, highlighting the importance of sleep in managing the condition and discussing strategies for improving sleep quality.

Sleep Patterns and Bipolar Disorder:

Individuals with bipolar disorder often experience disrupted sleep patterns characterized by insomnia, hypersomnia, or irregular sleep, wake cycles. During manic episodes, sleep may be significantly reduced, while depressive episodes may lead to excessive sleep. These disruptions can worsen mood symptoms and contribute to the cycling nature of bipolar disorder.

Sleep and Mood Regulation:

Sleep and mood regulation are closely interconnected. Sleep disturbances can trigger or exacerbate mood episodes in individuals with bipolar disorder. Sleep deprivation, for instance, has been linked to the onset of manic episodes. Conversely, a lack of restorative sleep can prolong depressive symptoms. Establishing healthy sleep patterns is crucial in stabilizing mood and managing the condition effectively.

Circadian Rhythm and Bipolar Disorder:

The circadian rhythm, our internal biological clock, plays a vital role in regulating sleep, wake cycles and maintaining overall health. Disruptions in the circadian rhythm have been observed in individuals with bipolar disorder. Irregular sleep schedules, such as irregular bedtimes or frequent changes in sleep patterns, can disrupt the circadian rhythm and contribute to mood instability. Maintaining a consistent sleep routine can help regulate the circadian rhythm and stabilize mood.

Sleep Medications and Treatment:

In the treatment of bipolar disorder, medications are often prescribed to manage symptoms and promote stability. Some of these medications, such as mood stabilizers or antipsychotics, may have sedating effects that can aid in improving sleep quality. However, careful monitoring and consultation with healthcare professionals are necessary to balance the benefits and potential side effects of sleep medications.

Sleep Hygiene Practices:

Adopting good sleep hygiene practices is crucial for individuals with bipolar disorder. This includes creating a sleep, conducive environment, maintaining a regular sleep schedule, and establishing a relaxing pre, sleep routine. Avoiding stimulants like caffeine or electronic devices before bedtime and ensuring a comfortable sleep environment can promote better sleep quality.

Cognitive Behavioral Therapy for Insomnia (CBT, I):

Cognitive Behavioral Therapy for Insomnia (CBT, I) is an evidence, based therapy that addresses the psychological and behavioral factors contributing to sleep disturbances. CBT, I techniques aim to improve sleep quality by challenging negative thoughts about sleep, implementing relaxation techniques, and establishing healthy sleep habits. Incorporating CBT, I into the treatment plan can have positive effects on sleep and overall well, being for individuals with bipolar disorder.

Light Therapy:

Light therapy, also known as phototherapy, is a non, invasive treatment approach that involves exposure to bright light to regulate circadian rhythms. It has been shown to be beneficial in managing mood symptoms in individuals with bipolar disorder, particularly those experiencing seasonal affective disorder (SAD). Light therapy can help regulate sleep patterns, improve mood, and mitigate the impact of seasonal variations on bipolar symptoms.

Monitoring and Tracking Sleep Patterns:

Keeping a sleep diary or using sleep, tracking apps can help individuals with bipolar disorder monitor their sleep patterns and identify any disturbances or trends. This information can be valuable in working with healthcare professionals to develop targeted interventions and treatment plans tailored to the individual's specific sleep needs.

The relationship between sleep and mood episodes

The Complex Interplay Between Sleep and Mood Episodes in Bipolar Disorder

Sleep and mood are intricately connected, and disruptions in sleep patterns can significantly impact individuals with bipolar disorder. This essay explores the complex relationship between sleep and mood episodes in bipolar disorder, shedding light on how sleep disturbances can influence the onset and severity of manic and depressive episodes.

Sleep Deprivation and Manic Episodes:

Sleep deprivation is often associated with the onset of manic episodes in individuals with bipolar disorder. Studies have shown that even a single night of sleep deprivation can trigger hypomanic or manic symptoms. Sleep loss affects brain functioning, leading to increased impulsivity, racing thoughts, and heightened energy levels. Recognizing the role of sleep deprivation in manic episodes is crucial for managing bipolar disorder effectively.

Sleep and Depressive Episodes:

While sleep deprivation is linked to manic episodes, disrupted sleep patterns can also exacerbate depressive symptoms in bipolar disorder. Insomnia or hypersomnia, which can occur during depressive episodes, contribute to low energy levels, fatigue, and a sense of hopelessness. Poor sleep quality can prolong and intensify depressive episodes, making effective sleep management essential for mood stabilization.

Circadian Rhythm Dysregulation:

Individuals with bipolar disorder often experience disruptions in their circadian rhythm, the internal biological clock regulating sleep, wake cycles. Irregular sleep patterns, such as late bedtimes or frequent changes in sleep schedules, can disrupt the circadian rhythm and contribute to mood instability. The dysregulation of the circadian rhythm further highlights the importance of maintaining consistent sleep routines for individuals with bipolar disorder.

Sleep Medications and Mood Stabilization:

Medications commonly prescribed for bipolar disorder, such as mood stabilizers and antipsychotics, may have sedating effects that help regulate sleep patterns. These medications can aid in stabilizing mood and reducing the frequency and severity of mood episodes. However, finding the right balance between medication, induced sedation and managing other side effects is crucial and should be done under the guidance of healthcare professionals.

Sleep Disturbances as Warning Signs:

Monitoring changes in sleep patterns can serve as an early warning system for impending mood episodes. Disruptions in sleep, such as insomnia, increased sleep duration, or irregular sleep, wake cycles, can signal an impending manic or depressive episode. Recognizing these patterns allows individuals to seek appropriate support and implement preventive strategies to minimize the impact of mood episodes.

Sleep Hygiene and Bipolar Disorder:

Establishing good sleep hygiene practices is vital for individuals with bipolar disorder. Maintaining a consistent sleep schedule, creating a calming sleep environment, and practicing relaxation techniques before bedtime can promote better sleep quality. Avoiding stimulants, such as caffeine or electronic devices, close to bedtime is also essential. Implementing these practices can contribute to better mood regulation and overall well, being.

Treating Sleep Disorders Concurrently:

It is not uncommon for individuals with bipolar disorder to experience comorbid sleep disorders, such as insomnia or sleep apnea. Treating these sleep disorders concurrently with bipolar disorder is crucial for optimal management. Addressing underlying sleep disturbances can have a positive impact on mood stability and overall functioning.

Collaborative Approach to Sleep Management:

Collaboration between individuals with bipolar disorder, healthcare professionals, and support networks is key in managing sleep disturbances and mood episodes effectively. Open communication, shared decision, making, and regular monitoring of sleep patterns can help tailor interventions and treatment plans to the individual's specific needs.

Sleep disorders associated with bipolar disorder

Unraveling the Relationship Between Sleep Disorders and Bipolar Disorder

Sleep disorders are commonly associated with bipolar disorder, and their presence can significantly impact the course and management of the condition. This essay explores the various sleep disorders that frequently co, occur with bipolar disorder, shedding light on their symptoms, implications, and the importance of addressing them in the context of bipolar disorder.

Insomnia and Bipolar Disorder:

Insomnia, characterized by difficulty falling asleep or staying asleep, is a prevalent sleep disorder among individuals with bipolar disorder. It can manifest during both manic and depressive episodes. Sleep disturbances associated with insomnia can worsen mood symptoms, impair daily functioning, and contribute to the cycling nature of bipolar disorder. Addressing insomnia is crucial for managing bipolar disorder effectively.

Hypersomnia and Bipolar Disorder:

Hypersomnia, excessive sleepiness or prolonged sleep duration, is another sleep disorder frequently observed in individuals with bipolar disorder, particularly during depressive episodes. Excessive sleep can further exacerbate depressive symptoms, hinder daily activities, and reduce overall productivity. Identifying and addressing hypersomnia is essential for improving quality of life and mood stability.

Circadian Rhythm Disorders and Bipolar Disorder:

Disruptions in the circadian rhythm, the internal biological clock regulating sleep, wake cycles, are commonly observed in bipolar disorder. Delayed sleep phase disorder (DSPD), where individuals have difficulty falling asleep and waking up at desired times, is prevalent among individuals with bipolar disorder. Irregular sleep, wake patterns and difficulties adapting to societal schedules can exacerbate mood instability. Strategies to regulate the circadian rhythm, such as light therapy and consistent sleep schedules, can help manage these disruptions.

Sleep Apnea and Bipolar Disorder:

Sleep apnea, characterized by interruptions in breathing during sleep, has been found to be more prevalent in individuals with bipolar disorder compared to the general population. The co, occurrence of sleep apnea can exacerbate mood symptoms, impair cognitive function, and contribute to overall health risks. Identifying and treating sleep apnea is crucial for optimizing treatment outcomes and overall well, being.

Restless Legs Syndrome and Bipolar Disorder:

Restless Legs Syndrome (RLS), characterized by an irresistible urge to move the legs during rest, is another sleep disorder commonly associated with bipolar disorder. RLS can lead to fragmented sleep, reduced sleep quality, and increased daytime fatigue. Managing RLS symptoms, which may involve medication and lifestyle modifications, can improve sleep and overall functioning in individuals with bipolar disorder.

Comorbid Substance Use and Sleep Disorders:

Substance use disorders frequently co, occur with bipolar disorder and can further complicate sleep disturbances. Substance abuse can disrupt sleep patterns, exacerbate mood symptoms, and hinder treatment outcomes. Addressing comorbid substance use disorders is essential for effectively managing both bipolar disorder and associated sleep disorders.

Impact of Sleep Disorders on Bipolar Treatment:

Sleep disorders can significantly impact the treatment of bipolar disorder. Disrupted sleep can affect medication response, reduce the effectiveness of therapy, and hinder the stability of mood episodes. Addressing sleep disorders alongside bipolar disorder treatment can enhance treatment outcomes and improve overall well, being.

Treatment Approaches for Sleep Disorders:

Treating sleep disorders in the context of bipolar disorder requires a multifaceted approach. Pharmacological interventions, such as sleep aids or mood stabilizers, may be prescribed to manage sleep disturbances. Non, pharmacological approaches, including cognitive, behavioral therapy for insomnia (CBT, I), sleep hygiene education, and relaxation techniques, can also be beneficial. A tailored approach that considers individual needs and preferences is essential for effective management.

Strategies for improving sleep hygiene and quality

Enhancing Sleep Hygiene and Quality: Strategies for Individuals with Bipolar Disorder

Establishing healthy sleep hygiene practices is essential for individuals with bipolar disorder to improve sleep quality and enhance overall well, being.

This essay explores effective strategies for enhancing sleep hygiene and promoting better sleep quality in the context of bipolar disorder, with the aim of stabilizing mood and optimizing treatment outcomes.

Establish Consistent Sleep Schedule:

Maintaining a consistent sleep schedule is crucial for regulating the circadian rhythm and promoting better sleep quality. Going to bed and waking up at the same time every day, including weekends, helps synchronize the body's internal clock and improves sleep efficiency. Establishing a regular sleep routine is particularly important for individuals with bipolar disorder to support mood stability.

Create a Sleep, Conducive Environment:

Creating a sleep, conducive environment can enhance relaxation and facilitate better sleep. Ensure the bedroom is cool, dark, and quiet, using curtains or blinds to block out excess light and reducing noise disturbances. Investing in a comfortable mattress, pillows, and bedding can also contribute to a more restful sleep experience.

Implement Relaxation Techniques:

Engaging in relaxation techniques before bedtime can help prepare the mind and body for sleep. Activities such as deep breathing exercises, progressive muscle relaxation, guided imagery, or meditation can promote a sense of calmness and relaxation. Incorporating these techniques into a nightly routine can signal the body to unwind and facilitate a smoother transition into sleep.

Limit Stimulants:

Avoiding stimulants, such as caffeine, nicotine, and alcohol, close to bedtime is essential for promoting better sleep quality. Stimulants can interfere with sleep onset and disrupt the overall sleep architecture. It is advisable to avoid consuming these substances several hours before bedtime to allow the body to wind down naturally.

Establish a Pre, Sleep Routine:

Engaging in a consistent pre, sleep routine can signal the body that it is time to prepare for sleep. This routine can include activities that promote relaxation and a sense of calm, such as reading a book, taking a warm bath, or listening to soothing music. Establishing a pre, sleep routine helps create a transition period between wakefulness and sleep, preparing the mind and body for restorative sleep.

Limit Exposure to Electronic Devices:

The blue light emitted by electronic devices, such as smartphones, tablets, and computers, can disrupt the body's natural sleep, wake cycle. It is recommended to avoid using electronic devices for at least one hour before bedtime. If necessary, using blue light filters or enabling night mode settings can help reduce the impact of electronic device usage on sleep quality.

Regular Physical Activity:

Engaging in regular physical activity has been shown to improve sleep quality and overall well, being. Incorporating moderate, intensity exercise, such as walking, jogging, or yoga, into daily routines can help regulate sleep patterns and promote a deeper and more restful sleep. However, it is important to avoid vigorous exercise close to bedtime, as it can stimulate the body and make it harder to fall asleep.

Manage Stress and Anxiety:

Stress and anxiety can significantly impact sleep quality. Developing effective stress management techniques, such as practicing mindfulness, engaging in relaxation exercises, or seeking support from therapists or support groups, can help alleviate anxiety and promote better sleep. It is important to establish a healthy coping mechanism for managing stressors associated with bipolar disorder.

Cognitive, Behavioral Therapy for Insomnia (CBT, I):

Cognitive, Behavioral Therapy for Insomnia (CBT, I) is a structured therapy that focuses on identifying and modifying negative thoughts and behaviors that contribute to insomnia. CBT, I helps individuals develop healthier sleep habits, challenge unhelpful beliefs about sleep, and implement strategies to improve sleep quality.

Chapter Twenty-Four

Bipolar Disorder and Nutrition

The Role of Nutrition in Managing Bipolar Disorder

Proper nutrition plays a crucial role in supporting overall health and well, being, including for individuals with bipolar disorder. While diet alone cannot treat the condition, adopting a healthy and balanced eating plan can contribute to mood stability, improve treatment outcomes, and enhance overall quality of life. This essay explores the relationship between bipolar disorder and nutrition, highlighting key dietary considerations and strategies for managing the condition effectively.

The Impact of Diet on Mood:

Emerging research suggests that certain dietary patterns can influence mood and mental health. Nutrient deficiencies or imbalances may affect neurotransmitter production and signaling, potentially exacerbating mood symptoms in individuals with bipolar disorder. A well, rounded diet that provides essential nutrients can support brain function and contribute to mood stability.

Balancing Macronutrients:

Balancing macronutrients—carbohydrates, proteins, and fats—is important for individuals with bipolar disorder. Consuming complex carbohydrates, such as whole grains, fruits, and vegetables, helps regulate blood sugar levels and provide a steady source of energy. Including lean proteins and healthy fats, such as fish, nuts, and avocados, can support brain health and mood regulation.

Omega, 3 Fatty Acids:

Omega, 3 fatty acids, found in fatty fish like salmon, sardines, and mackerel, have been associated with improved mental health outcomes. These essential fatty acids play a role in brain function and have anti, inflammatory properties that may benefit individuals with bipolar disorder. Incorporating omega, 3, rich foods or considering supplements can be beneficial, but consultation with healthcare professionals is advised.

Micronutrient Considerations:

Certain vitamins and minerals play a vital role in brain health and mood regulation. For example, studies have shown a potential link between low levels of B vitamins, including folate and vitamin B12, and increased risk of mood disorders. Including sources of these nutrients, such as leafy greens, legumes, and fortified cereals, can support overall well, being.

Gut, Brain Connection:

The gut microbiome, the diverse community of bacteria residing in the digestive system, has been increasingly recognized for its influence on mental health. Research suggests that imbalances in the gut microbiota may contribute to mood disturbances. Consuming a diet rich in fiber, fermented foods (e.g., yogurt, sauerkraut), and prebiotic, rich foods (e.g., garlic, onions) can support a healthy gut microbiome and potentially positively impact mood.

Caffeine and Alcohol:

Caffeine and alcohol consumption can significantly affect individuals with bipolar disorder. Caffeine, found in coffee, tea, and energy drinks, is a stimulant that can disrupt sleep, exacerbate anxiety, and potentially trigger manic episodes. Alcohol, on the other hand, can interact with medications and destabilize mood. Limiting or avoiding these substances is advisable for better symptom management.

Meal Regularity and Stability:

Maintaining regular meal times and avoiding long periods without eating can help stabilize blood sugar levels and support mood regulation. Irregular eating patterns or skipping meals can contribute to mood swings and energy fluctuations. Planning and preparing meals in advance, incorporating a variety of nutrient, rich foods, and having regular meal times can promote stability.

Working with a Registered Dietitian:

Working with a registered dietitian experienced in mental health and nutrition can be valuable for individuals with bipolar disorder. A dietitian can provide personalized guidance, develop meal plans, and address specific nutritional concerns or restrictions. They can also help navigate medication interactions and ensure nutrient adequacy.

The role of diet in managing mood and overall health

Diet plays a fundamental role in maintaining overall health and well, being. Emerging research suggests that the foods we consume can impact our mood, mental health, and overall quality of life. For individuals with bipolar disorder, a healthy diet can be particularly beneficial in managing mood symptoms and supporting treatment. This essay explores the role of diet in managing mood and overall health, with a specific focus on its relevance to individuals with bipolar disorder.

The Gut, Brain Connection:

The gut, brain connection refers to the bidirectional communication between the digestive system and the brain. Research indicates that the gut microbiome, the complex community of microorganisms in the gut, can influence mood, cognition, and behavior. A diet rich in fiber, fruits, vegetables, and fermented foods promotes a healthy gut microbiome, which may contribute to better mental health outcomes.

Balanced Macronutrients:

Balancing macronutrients, including carbohydrates, proteins, and fats, is essential for stable energy levels and optimal brain function. Complex carbohydrates, such as whole grains, legumes, and vegetables, provide a steady release of glucose, supporting mood stability. Lean proteins, like poultry, fish, and tofu, supply amino acids necessary for neurotransmitter synthesis. Healthy fats, such as avocados, nuts, and olive oil, are crucial for brain health and mood regulation.

Nutrient, Rich Foods:

Consuming a variety of nutrient, rich foods provides essential vitamins, minerals, and antioxidants. B vitamins, including folate, vitamin B12, and vitamin B6, are particularly important for mental health. Leafy greens, legumes, eggs, and fortified cereals are excellent sources of these nutrients. Antioxidant, rich foods, such as berries, dark chocolate, and green tea, help reduce inflammation and oxidative stress, potentially benefiting mood regulation.

Omega, 3 Fatty Acids:

Omega, 3 fatty acids, especially eicosapentaenoic acid (EPA) and docosahexaenoic acid (DHA), have been associated with improved mood and cognitive function. Fatty fish, such as salmon, mackerel, and sardines, are excellent sources of omega, 3 fatty acids. Vegetarian sources include flaxseeds, chia seeds, and walnuts. Incorporating these foods into the diet or considering omega, 3 supplements may be beneficial for individuals with bipolar disorder.

Caffeine and Sugar:

While caffeine can provide a temporary energy boost, excessive consumption can disrupt sleep patterns and exacerbate anxiety and irritability. Individuals with bipolar disorder should be cautious about their caffeine intake and consider switching to decaffeinated options or herbal teas. Similarly, excessive sugar consumption can lead to energy fluctuations and mood swings. Opting for natural sweeteners or reducing sugar intake can help stabilize mood and energy levels.

Mindful Eating:

Practicing mindful eating involves paying attention to the sensory experience of eating and tuning into hunger and satiety cues. This approach promotes a healthier relationship with food and helps prevent overeating or emotional eating, which can affect mood and overall well, being. Engaging in mindful eating techniques, such as eating slowly, savoring flavors, and listening to internal hunger cues, can enhance the enjoyment and nutritional value of meals.

Hydration:

Proper hydration is essential for optimal brain function and overall health. Dehydration can contribute to fatigue, mood changes, and cognitive impairment. Ensuring an adequate intake of water throughout the day is vital. Herbal teas, infused water, and consuming water, rich foods like fruits and vegetables are excellent ways to stay hydrated.

Nutritional deficiencies and supplementation

Uncovering Nutritional Deficiencies and Supplementation in Bipolar Disorder

Nutritional deficiencies can have a profound impact on overall health, including mental well, being. For individuals with bipolar disorder, addressing potential nutrient imbalances is crucial as they may contribute to mood fluctuations and treatment outcomes. This essay explores the connection between nutritional deficiencies and bipolar disorder, highlighting key nutrients, their impact on mental health, and the role of supplementation in managing the condition effectively.

Vitamin D:

Vitamin D plays a vital role in brain health and mood regulation. Deficiencies in this vitamin have been associated with an increased risk of mood disorders, including bipolar disorder. Sun exposure and certain foods like fatty fish, fortified dairy products, and eggs are natural sources of vitamin D. However, supplementation may be necessary, particularly in individuals with limited sun exposure or inadequate dietary intake.

B Vitamins:

B vitamins, including folate, vitamin B12, and vitamin B6, are essential for brain function and neurotransmitter synthesis. Deficiencies in these vitamins have been linked to an increased risk of mood disorders. Leafy greens, legumes, fortified cereals, poultry, and fish are excellent dietary sources. In some cases, supplementation or increased intake through fortified foods may be recommended.

Omega, 3 Fatty Acids:

Omega, 3 fatty acids, specifically EPA and DHA, have been studied extensively for their positive effects on mental health. They contribute to brain structure and function, promote anti, inflammatory processes, and support mood regulation. Fatty fish, flaxseeds, chia seeds, and walnuts are natural sources. For individuals with bipolar disorder, omega, 3 fatty acid supplementation may be considered to ensure adequate intake.

Minerals:

Mineral deficiencies can impact mental health and exacerbate mood symptoms in individuals with bipolar disorder. Zinc, magnesium, and iron are particularly relevant. Zinc plays a role in neurotransmitter function and is found in foods like oysters, beef, and legumes. Magnesium, present in leafy greens, nuts, and whole grains, is involved in stress management and relaxation. Iron deficiency can lead to fatigue and low mood and can be addressed through iron, rich foods like lean meats, beans, and fortified grains.

Antioxidants:

Antioxidants protect the brain from oxidative stress and inflammation, which can contribute to mood disorders. Vitamin C, vitamin E, and selenium are notable antioxidants. Citrus fruits, berries, nuts, and seeds are rich in vitamin C and E. Selenium is found in Brazil nuts, seafood, and whole grains. A diet abundant in fruits, vegetables, and whole foods provides a range of antioxidants.

Considerations for Supplementation:

Supplementation should be approached cautiously and under the guidance of healthcare professionals. Comprehensive blood testing can help identify specific nutrient deficiencies, ensuring targeted supplementation. Working with a registered dietitian or a healthcare provider knowledgeable in mental health and nutrition can help determine appropriate supplement dosages and monitor their efficacy.

Individualized Approach:

Nutritional needs are highly individual, and it is essential to consider personal factors, such as age, sex, lifestyle, and any underlying health conditions, when addressing nutritional deficiencies. An individualized approach that considers dietary preferences, cultural practices, and potential interactions with medications is crucial for success.

The Importance of a Balanced Diet:

While supplementation can be beneficial, it is essential to prioritize a balanced diet as the foundation of nutritional well, being. Whole foods, including fruits, vegetables, lean proteins, whole grains, and healthy fats, provide a variety of essential nutrients. Focusing on nutrient, dense meals and snacks ensures a broad spectrum of vitamins, minerals, and antioxidants.

Developing a balanced and sustainable eating plan

Nurturing Balance: Developing a Balanced and Sustainable Eating Plan for Bipolar Disorder

Developing a balanced and sustainable eating plan is essential for individuals with bipolar disorder to support overall well, being and manage mood symptoms. A nourishing diet can provide the necessary nutrients, stabilize blood sugar levels, and promote stable energy throughout the day. This essay explores the key principles of developing a balanced and sustainable eating plan in the context of bipolar disorder, emphasizing the importance of nourishment, variety, and long, term sustainability.

Emphasize Nutrient, Dense Foods:

A balanced eating plan for bipolar disorder should prioritize nutrient, dense foods that provide essential vitamins, minerals, and antioxidants. Incorporate a variety of fruits, vegetables, whole grains, lean proteins, and healthy fats into daily meals. These foods not only nourish the body but also contribute to overall mental well, being.

Include Complex Carbohydrates:

Complex carbohydrates are a valuable source of energy and promote stable blood sugar levels. Whole grains, legumes, fruits, and vegetables are excellent sources of complex carbohydrates. These foods provide a sustained release of energy and support mood stability.

Opt for Lean Proteins:

Including lean proteins in the diet helps maintain satiety, stabilize blood sugar levels, and support neurotransmitter synthesis. Choose lean sources such as poultry, fish, legumes, tofu, and Greek yogurt. These proteins are rich in essential amino acids necessary for optimal brain function.

Healthy Fats for Brain Health:

Incorporating healthy fats is essential for brain health and mood regulation. Include sources such as avocados, nuts, seeds, olive oil, and fatty fish (rich in omega, 3 fatty acids). These fats provide essential nutrients, promote satiety, and support cognitive function.

Prioritize Plant, Based Foods:

A plant, focused eating plan can provide an abundance of nutrients, antioxidants, and fiber. Aim to incorporate a variety of fruits, vegetables, whole grains, legumes, nuts, and seeds. Plant, based foods are rich in phytonutrients that support brain health and reduce inflammation.

Moderation and Mindful Eating:

Adopting a mindful eating approach encourages awareness of hunger and fullness cues and promotes a balanced relationship with food. Practice portion control, savor each bite, and listen to your body's signals. Avoid restrictive diets or labeling foods as "good" or "bad," as they can lead to unhealthy relationships with food.

Hydration for Optimal Functioning:

Proper hydration is crucial for optimal brain function and overall health. Aim to drink an adequate amount of water throughout the day. Hydrating foods, such as fruits and vegetables, also contribute to overall hydration levels.

Meal Planning and Preparation:

Developing a balanced eating plan is facilitated by meal planning and preparation. Plan meals ahead of time, incorporate a variety of food groups, and consider batch cooking to ensure convenient access to nourishing meals throughout the week. Having healthy options readily available reduces the likelihood of turning to less nutritious choices.

Individualized Approach:

Recognize that individual nutritional needs may vary based on factors such as age, sex, activity level, and personal preferences. Tailor the eating plan to suit your specific requirements and lifestyle. Consulting with a registered dietitian or nutritionist who specializes in bipolar disorder can provide personalized guidance.

Long, Term Sustainability:

Focus on developing an eating plan that is sustainable in the long term. Avoid quick, fix diets or extreme restrictions that can be challenging to maintain. Instead, aim for a balanced approach that integrates enjoyable and nourishing foods, allowing for flexibility and enjoyment while still meeting nutritional needs.

Chapter Twenty-Five

Bipolar Disorder and Physical Activity

Empowering Stability: The Role of Physical Activity in Bipolar Disorder

Physical activity is a powerful tool in managing bipolar disorder, promoting overall well, being, and enhancing treatment outcomes. Regular exercise has been shown to alleviate mood symptoms, reduce stress, improve sleep, and enhance overall quality of life. This essay explores the relationship between bipolar disorder and physical activity, highlighting its benefits, considerations, and strategies for incorporating exercise into a bipolar management plan.

Mood Regulation through Exercise:

Physical activity has a direct impact on mood regulation and can effectively complement other treatment modalities for bipolar disorder. Exercise stimulates the release of endorphins, neurotransmitters that elevate mood and promote a sense of well, being. Engaging in regular exercise can help reduce symptoms of depression and anxiety, stabilize mood, and promote emotional balance.

Stress Reduction and Coping Mechanisms:

Stress is a common trigger for mood episodes in individuals with bipolar disorder. Regular physical activity serves as a natural stress reducer by lowering cortisol levels, improving cardiovascular health, and promoting relaxation. Exercise also offers an opportunity to develop healthy coping mechanisms, providing a constructive outlet for managing stressors associated with bipolar disorder.

Sleep Quality and Regulation:

Sleep disturbances are prevalent in bipolar disorder and can significantly impact mood stability. Regular physical activity can improve sleep quality, reduce insomnia symptoms, and regulate sleep patterns. Engaging in exercise during the day can promote a more restful night's sleep, contributing to overall well, being and mood regulation.

Neuroplasticity and Cognitive Function:

Bipolar disorder affects cognitive function, including memory, attention, and executive functioning. Physical activity has been shown to enhance neuroplasticity, the brain's ability to adapt and form new neural connections. Regular exercise supports cognitive health, improving memory, concentration, and overall cognitive function in individuals with bipolar disorder.

Considerations for Physical Activity:

When incorporating physical activity into a bipolar management plan, it is important to consider individual needs, preferences, and any physical limitations. Consulting with healthcare professionals, including psychiatrists and physical therapists, can help develop an exercise routine tailored to the individual's capabilities and specific mental health needs.

Finding the Right Type of Exercise:

The type of exercise chosen should align with individual preferences and physical abilities. Options may include aerobic exercises (e.g., brisk walking, swimming, cycling) that elevate heart rate and promote cardiovascular health, as well as activities such as yoga, tai chi, or Pilates, which emphasize mindfulness and relaxation. Experimenting with different forms of exercise can help identify enjoyable and sustainable options.

Establishing a Routine:

Consistency is key when it comes to reaping the benefits of physical activity. Establishing a regular exercise routine, aiming for at least 150 minutes of moderate, intensity aerobic activity per week, promotes adherence and maximizes the positive impact on mood and overall well, being. Breaking exercise sessions into shorter, more manageable intervals can be beneficial for individuals with fluctuating energy levels.

Social Support and Accountability:

Engaging in physical activity with others can provide social support and enhance motivation. Joining group fitness classes, participating in team sports, or finding an exercise buddy can foster a sense of community and accountability. It also offers opportunities for social interaction, reducing feelings of isolation often experienced by individuals with bipolar disorder.

Gradual Progression and Self, Compassion:

When starting or returning to an exercise routine, it is important to practice self, compassion and allow for gradual progression. Start with low, impact activities and gradually increase intensity and duration as fitness levels improve. Setting realistic goals and celebrating small achievements can help maintain motivation and prevent setbacks.

The benefits of exercise for mental health

Unleashing the Power Within: The Transformative Benefits of Exercise for Mental Health

Exercise is a potent ally in promoting mental health and well, being, with its positive impact reaching far beyond physical fitness. In the realm of bipolar disorder, exercise holds immense potential as a complementary therapy for managing mood symptoms and enhancing overall mental wellness. This essay explores the benefits of exercise for mental health, highlighting its relevance in the context of bipolar disorders, and emphasizing its transformative effects on the mind and body.

Mood Elevation and Emotional Well, being:

Exercise has a direct impact on mood elevation, triggering the release of endorphins—natural mood, enhancing chemicals—in the brain. These endorphins promote feelings of happiness, reduce stress and anxiety, and enhance overall emotional well, being. Regular exercise can be particularly advantageous for individuals with bipolar disorder, helping to stabilize mood, minimize depressive symptoms, and alleviate anxiety.

Stress Reduction and Resilience Building:

Physical activity is a powerful stress, reduction tool, offering a healthy outlet for managing and coping with stress. Engaging in exercise helps reduce cortisol levels—the primary stress hormone—and triggers the release of feel, good neurotransmitters, such as serotonin and dopamine. Regular exercise can enhance resilience, improve stress management skills, and reduce the risk of mood episodes associated with bipolar disorder.

Cognitive Function and Mental Sharpness:

Exercise has a profound impact on cognitive function, including memory, attention, and executive functioning. Aerobic exercise, in particular, promotes blood flow to the brain, which enhances neuroplasticity—the brain's ability to form new connections—and supports cognitive performance. By engaging in regular exercise, individuals with bipolar disorder can improve mental sharpness, memory retention, and overall cognitive function.

Sleep Quality and Regulation:

Sleep disturbances are common in bipolar disorder and can significantly impact mood stability. Regular exercise has been shown to improve sleep quality, promote deeper and more restful sleep, and regulate sleep patterns. By incorporating physical activity into their routine, individuals with bipolar disorder can enhance their sleep quality, which, in turn, positively influences mood, energy levels, and overall well, being.

Self, esteem and Body Image:

Exercise can have a transformative impact on self, esteem and body image. Regular physical activity helps individuals feel more confident, capable, and empowered. Achieving personal fitness goals, improving physical fitness, and experiencing the positive changes in their body can enhance self, esteem and body image. For individuals with bipolar disorder, exercise can be a powerful tool for fostering a positive self, perception and cultivating a sense of self, worth.

Social Connection and Support:

Engaging in exercise often provides opportunities for social connection and support, which are vital components of mental health. Joining group fitness classes, participating in team sports, or engaging in outdoor activities with others can foster a sense of community, reduce social isolation, and enhance overall well, being. The social aspect of exercise can be particularly beneficial for individuals with bipolar disorder, as it combats loneliness and creates a supportive network.

Medication Complement and Treatment Enhancement:

Exercise should be seen as a complement to, rather than a replacement for, medication and other treatment modalities for bipolar disorder. Regular physical activity can enhance the effectiveness of medication, optimize treatment outcomes, and reduce the reliance on medication alone. It is important to consult with healthcare professionals to determine the most appropriate exercise plan that aligns with individual needs and treatment goals.

Incorporating Exercise into Daily Life:

Integrating exercise into daily life is essential for reaping the full benefits. Finding activities that are enjoyable, sustainable, and align with personal preferences is crucial. Whether it's walking, jogging, dancing, swimming, or engaging in sports, the key is to engage in physical activity consistently.

Choosing the right type and intensity of exercise

Finding Your Fit: Choosing the Right Type and Intensity of Exercise for Bipolar Disorder

When it comes to exercise, finding the right type and intensity is crucial for individuals with bipolar disorder. Different forms of exercise offer unique benefits and considerations, and tailoring physical activity to individual needs is essential for maximizing the positive impact on mood, overall well, being, and managing bipolar symptoms. This essay explores the factors to consider when choosing the right type and intensity of exercise in the context of bipolar disorder, emphasizing the importance of personal preferences, physical capabilities, and mental health considerations.

Consider Personal Preferences:

Choosing an exercise routine that aligns with personal preferences is key to maintaining motivation and long, term adherence. Whether it's engaging in outdoor activities, joining a gym, dancing, swimming, or participating in team sports, finding activities that are enjoyable and bring a sense of fulfillment enhances the overall exercise experience and increases the likelihood of continued engagement.

Assess Physical Capabilities:

Taking into account individual physical capabilities and any specific health concerns is crucial when selecting the right type and intensity of exercise. Consulting with healthcare professionals, such as a primary care physician or physical therapist, can provide insights into any potential limitations or modifications that may be necessary. Considering factors such as age, fitness level, and any existing injuries or health conditions ensures exercise is safe and suitable.

Aerobic Exercise for Mood Stability:

Aerobic exercise, such as brisk walking, jogging, cycling, or swimming, has been shown to have significant mood, stabilizing effects. It increases the release of endorphins, improves cardiovascular health, and enhances brain function. Engaging in moderate, intensity aerobic activities for at least 150 minutes per week can positively impact mood, reduce depressive symptoms, and contribute to overall well, being.

Strength Training for Empowerment:

Strength training, involving resistance exercises using weights, resistance bands, or bodyweight, offers unique benefits for individuals with bipolar disorder. It enhances muscular strength, improves bone health, and supports overall functional capacity. Strength training can foster a sense of empowerment and accomplishment, boosting self, esteem and resilience in managing bipolar symptoms.

Mind, Body Practices for Stress Reduction:

Mind, body practices, such as yoga, tai chi, and Pilates, combine physical movement with mindfulness and relaxation techniques. These practices offer gentle yet effective ways to reduce stress, enhance body awareness, and promote mental calmness. Mind, body exercises can help individuals with bipolar disorder manage anxiety, improve sleep quality, and cultivate a greater sense of overall well, being.

Interval Training for Energy and Motivation:

Interval training, which involves alternating periods of high, intensity exercise with recovery periods, can be a time, efficient and energizing option. It boosts cardiovascular fitness, enhances metabolic function, and improves mood. Incorporating short bursts of high, intensity activity, such as sprinting, jumping jacks, or cycling, followed by recovery periods, can provide a challenging yet rewarding exercise experience.

Outdoor Activities for Connection with Nature:

Engaging in outdoor activities, such as hiking, gardening, or participating in team sports, offers the added benefits of connecting with nature and enjoying fresh air. Outdoor exercise promotes mental relaxation, reduces stress, and enhances overall well, being. The sights, sounds, and natural surroundings can create a sense of serenity and provide a welcome escape from daily stressors.

Considerations for Energy Levels:

Individuals with bipolar disorder may experience fluctuations in energy levels. It is important to choose exercise types and intensities that align with these fluctuations. On days when energy levels are high, engaging in moderate to high, intensity activities can be invigorating. On low, energy days, opting for low, impact exercises, gentle stretching, or shorter durations of activity can still be beneficial.

Building a consistent and enjoyable fitness routine

Building Your Foundation: Creating a Consistent and Enjoyable Fitness Routine for Bipolar Disorder

Establishing a consistent and enjoyable fitness routine is essential for individuals with bipolar disorder to harness the transformative power of exercise. A well, rounded exercise regimen not only supports physical fitness but also plays a crucial role in managing mood symptoms and promoting overall well, being. This essay explores the key strategies for building a consistent and enjoyable fitness routine in the context of bipolar disorder, emphasizing the importance of individual preferences, goal setting, and self, care.

Identify Personal Preferences:

Finding activities that align with personal preferences is essential for creating a sustainable fitness routine. Reflect on the types of physical activities that bring joy and fulfillment. It may involve exploring various exercise modalities, such as dancing, swimming, hiking, or group fitness classes. By engaging in activities that are enjoyable, individuals with bipolar disorder are more likely to maintain long, term adherence to their fitness routine.

Set Realistic and Achievable Goals:

Setting realistic and achievable goals helps provide structure and motivation to the fitness routine. Begin by identifying specific goals related to physical fitness, mental health, or overall well, being. These goals can be as simple as committing to a certain number of weekly workouts, increasing daily step count, or improving flexibility. Celebrate milestones and use them as inspiration to maintain consistency.

Start Slow and Gradually Increase Intensity:

When beginning a fitness routine, it is important to start slow and gradually increase intensity. This approach helps prevent injuries, minimizes the risk of burnout, and allows the body to adapt to new physical demands. Begin with low, impact exercises, shorter durations, or lower intensity workouts, and gradually progress over time. Listening to the body's signals and adjusting intensity accordingly fosters a sustainable and enjoyable routine.

Incorporate Variety and Cross, Training:

Introducing variety and cross, training into the fitness routine offers numerous benefits. Not only does it prevent monotony and boredom, but it also engages different muscle groups, promotes overall fitness, and reduces the risk of overuse injuries. Mix up aerobic exercises, strength training, flexibility work, and mind, body practices. Engaging in different activities on different days keeps the routine fresh and exciting.

Establish a Consistent Schedule:

Consistency is key to reaping the benefits of exercise. Establish a regular schedule that allows for dedicated exercise time. Consistency fosters habit formation and ensures that exercise becomes an integral part of daily life. Block off specific time slots for workouts, treating them as non, negotiable commitments to one's well, being.

Prioritize Self, Care and Recovery:

Integrating self, care and recovery into the fitness routine is essential for individuals with bipolar disorder. Allow time for rest and recovery, especially after intense workouts. Practice self, care activities, such as stretching, foam rolling, or engaging in relaxation techniques like meditation or deep breathing. Balancing physical exertion with restorative practices supports optimal mental and physical health.

Seek Support and Accountability:

Seeking support and accountability can enhance motivation and adherence to a fitness routine. Consider enlisting a workout buddy, joining group fitness classes, or participating in online communities focused on exercise and mental health. These avenues provide opportunities for social interaction, encouragement, and the sharing of experiences with like, minded individuals.

Adapt to Fluctuating Energy Levels:

Individuals with bipolar disorder may experience fluctuations in energy levels. It is important to adapt the fitness routine to accommodate these changes. On days when energy levels are high, embrace higher, intensity workouts or longer durations. On low, energy days, opt for gentle exercises, shorter workouts, or focus on restorative practices like yoga or tai chi. Flexibility and adaptability allow for continued engagement in physical activity, regardless of energy fluctuations.

Chapter Twenty-Six

Alternative and Complementary Therapies

Expanding Horizons: Exploring Alternative and Complementary Therapies for Bipolar Disorder

In addition to traditional medical treatments, alternative and complementary therapies can offer valuable support for individuals with bipolar disorder. These therapies, which encompass a range of holistic approaches, can enhance overall well, being, complement existing treatments, and empower individuals in their journey toward stability. This essay explores various alternative and complementary therapies in the context of bipolar disorder, highlighting their potential benefits, considerations, and integration into a comprehensive treatment plan.

Mindfulness and Meditation:

Mindfulness and meditation practices cultivate present, moment awareness, promote relaxation, and reduce stress. These practices can be beneficial for individuals with bipolar disorder, helping to manage mood symptoms, improve emotional regulation, and increase self, awareness. Incorporating mindfulness and meditation into daily life, even for a few minutes a day, can support mental well, being.

Yoga and Tai Chi:

Yoga and Tai Chi are mind, body practices that combine movement, breathwork, and meditation. They promote physical strength, flexibility, and balance while fostering relaxation and emotional well, being. Regular practice of yoga or Tai Chi can reduce stress, enhance self, awareness, and improve mood stability. Modified poses and adaptations can accommodate physical limitations and ensure safety.

Acupuncture:

Acupuncture, an ancient Chinese therapy, involves the insertion of thin needles into specific points on the body to promote balance and restore energy flow. Research suggests that acupuncture may help reduce depressive symptoms and stabilize mood in individuals with bipolar disorder. Seeking a licensed and experienced acupuncturist is important to ensure safe and effective treatment.

Massage Therapy:

Massage therapy involves manual manipulation of soft tissues to promote relaxation and relieve muscle tension. It can reduce anxiety, improve sleep quality, and enhance overall well, being. Massage therapy may be beneficial for individuals with bipolar disorder, especially during depressive episodes, as it can provide comfort, relaxation, and a sense of nurturing.

Herbal and Nutritional Supplements:

Herbal and nutritional supplements are widely used as complementary approaches in mental health. Certain supplements, such as omega, 3 fatty acids, St. John's wort, and S, adenosylmethionine (SAMe), have shown promise in reducing depressive symptoms. However, it is crucial to consult with healthcare professionals before starting any supplements, as they can interact with medications and vary in effectiveness.

Light Therapy:

Light therapy involves exposure to bright, artificial light to simulate natural sunlight. It is commonly used to treat seasonal affective disorder (SAD) but may also benefit individuals with bipolar disorder experiencing depressive episodes. Light therapy can regulate circadian rhythms, improve mood, and enhance energy levels. Consulting with a healthcare professional can help determine the appropriate duration and intensity of light exposure.

Exercise and Physical Activity:

Regular exercise and physical activity are considered alternative therapies that have a profound impact on mental health. Engaging in aerobic exercises, strength training, or other forms of physical activity releases endorphins, reduces stress, and promotes overall well, being. Incorporating exercise into daily life can enhance mood stability, increase energy levels, and improve overall mental health.

Art Therapy:

Art therapy involves creative expression through various art forms, such as painting, drawing, or sculpting. It can provide a therapeutic outlet for individuals with bipolar disorder, facilitating self, expression, emotional processing, and stress reduction. Engaging in art therapy can enhance self, awareness, foster a sense of control, and promote emotional healing.

Music Therapy:

Music therapy utilizes music to support emotional and psychological well, being. Listening to or creating music can be a powerful medium for self, expression, relaxation, and mood modulation. Music therapy can reduce stress, improve mood, and serve as a coping mechanism for individuals with bipolar disorder.

Herbal remedies and dietary supplements

Nurturing Balance: Herbal Remedies and Dietary Supplements in Bipolar Disorder Management

Herbal remedies and dietary supplements have gained popularity as alternative approaches to support mental health and well, being. For individuals with bipolar disorder, exploring the potential benefits of these natural interventions can be of interest. However, it is essential to approach herbal remedies and dietary supplements with caution, considering their effectiveness, safety, and potential interactions with medications. This essay explores the use of herbal remedies and dietary supplements in the context of bipolar disorder management, providing insights into their potential benefits, considerations, and the importance of professional guidance.

St. John's Wort:

St. John's Wort is a herbal remedy commonly used for mood disorders, including depression. Some studies suggest that it may alleviate depressive symptoms in individuals with mild, to, moderate depression. However, its use in bipolar disorder is controversial due to the potential risk of triggering manic or hypomanic episodes. It is crucial to consult with a healthcare professional before considering St. John's Wort as a complementary treatment for bipolar disorder.

Omega, 3 Fatty Acids:

Omega, 3 fatty acids, primarily found in fatty fish like salmon and mackerel, as well as in plant, based sources such as flaxseeds and walnuts, have shown potential in supporting mental health. Research suggests that omega, 3 supplementation may help reduce depressive symptoms and promote overall well, being. While further investigation is needed, incorporating omega, 3 fatty acids into the diet or considering supplements under professional guidance may be beneficial for individuals with bipolar disorder.

S, adenosylmethionine (SAMe):

SAMe is a naturally occurring compound involved in various biochemical processes in the body, including neurotransmitter production. Some studies suggest that SAMe may be effective in reducing depressive symptoms. However, evidence specific to bipolar disorder is limited. SAMe can interact with certain medications, and its use should be discussed with a healthcare professional to determine safety, appropriate dosages, and potential benefits.

Rhodiola Rosea:

Rhodiola Rosea is an adaptogenic herb that has been traditionally used to combat stress and fatigue. It has shown promise in improving energy levels, reducing anxiety, and enhancing overall well, being. Although some studies suggest potential benefits in mood regulation, evidence specific to bipolar disorder is limited. Individuals with bipolar disorder should exercise caution, as rhodiola may trigger manic or hypomanic episodes. Consultation with a healthcare professional is advised.

Vitamin and Mineral Supplements:

Certain vitamins and minerals play a crucial role in mental health and may be deficient in individuals with bipolar disorder. These include vitamin D, B vitamins (particularly folate and vitamin B12), and minerals such as magnesium and zinc. Deficiencies in these nutrients can affect mood regulation and overall well, being. Assessing nutrient levels through blood tests and considering supplementation under professional guidance may be necessary to address specific deficiencies.

Herbal Teas:

Herbal teas, such as chamomile, lavender, and passionflower, are known for their calming properties and may help reduce anxiety and promote relaxation. While herbal teas do not typically pose significant risks or interactions, their effects on bipolar disorder symptoms are limited. Herbal teas can serve as a comforting and soothing beverage but should not replace prescribed medications or professional guidance.

Professional Guidance and Monitoring:

The use of herbal remedies and dietary supplements should be approached with caution and under professional guidance. Consulting with a healthcare professional, particularly a psychiatrist or a registered dietitian, is crucial to assess individual needs, potential interactions with medications, and appropriate dosages. Regular monitoring, including blood tests, can help evaluate the efficacy and safety of supplementation.

Acupuncture, massage, and other bodywork therapies

Balancing Body and Mind: Exploring Acupuncture, Massage, and Other Bodywork Therapies for Bipolar Disorder

In addition to traditional medical treatments, alternative therapies such as acupuncture, massage, and other bodywork techniques have gained recognition for their potential benefits in managing mental health conditions, including bipolar disorder. These therapies offer holistic approaches that aim to restore balance, reduce stress, and promote overall well, being. This essay explores the use of acupuncture, massage, and other bodywork therapies in the context of bipolar disorder, shedding light on their potential benefits, considerations, and integration into a comprehensive treatment plan.

Acupuncture:

Acupuncture is an ancient Chinese therapy involving the insertion of thin needles into specific points on the body. It aims to restore the flow of energy and rebalance the body. Although research on acupuncture for bipolar disorder is limited, some studies suggest potential benefits in reducing depressive symptoms and promoting emotional well, being. Acupuncture should be performed by a licensed and experienced practitioner who understands the complexities of bipolar disorder and can tailor treatments accordingly.

Massage Therapy:

Massage therapy involves manual manipulation of soft tissues to promote relaxation, reduce muscle tension, and improve overall well, being. Massage can enhance mood, alleviate anxiety, and provide a sense of nurturing and comfort. For individuals with bipolar disorder, massage therapy can serve as a complementary tool to manage stress, promote relaxation, and support overall mental health. Communication with the massage therapist about individual needs, preferences, and any specific considerations related to bipolar disorder is essential.

Craniosacral Therapy:

Craniosacral therapy is a gentle, hands, on approach that aims to enhance the functioning of the central nervous system. It involves applying light pressure and manipulations to the skull, spine, and pelvis. This therapy can promote relaxation, relieve tension, and restore balance in the body. While research specifically on craniosacral therapy for bipolar disorder is limited, it may be worth exploring as part of a comprehensive treatment plan. Consulting with a skilled practitioner who has experience working with mental health conditions is important.

Reiki:

Reiki is an energy, based healing technique that involves the gentle placement of hands on or above the body to channel healing energy. It aims to rebalance the body's energy and promote a sense of harmony and well, being. Reiki can induce relaxation, reduce stress, and support emotional healing. While research on Reiki for bipolar disorder is limited, it can be a complementary therapy to manage stress, enhance relaxation, and promote overall well, being. Seeking a certified Reiki practitioner who understands the complexities of bipolar disorder is crucial.

Reflexology:

Reflexology is a therapy that involves applying pressure to specific points on the feet, hands, or ears that correspond to various organs and systems in the body. It aims to promote relaxation, reduce tension, and restore balance. Reflexology can be a soothing and relaxing therapy for individuals with bipolar disorder. While there is limited research on its specific effects in bipolar disorder, it can be used as a complementary therapy to support overall mental well, being. Working with a trained reflexologist who is knowledgeable about bipolar disorder is important.

Aromatherapy:

Aromatherapy involves the use of essential oils derived from plants to promote relaxation, reduce anxiety, and support emotional well, being. Essential oils can be diffused, applied topically, or used in baths. While aromatherapy alone may not be a primary treatment for bipolar disorder, incorporating it into a self, care routine can provide relaxation and emotional support. It is important to choose high, quality essential oils, follow proper usage guidelines, and be mindful of individual sensitivities or allergies.

Art, music, and other creative therapies

Unleashing Creative Expression: Exploring Art, Music, and Other Creative Therapies for Bipolar Disorder

Creative therapies, such as art and music, offer unique avenues for self, expression, emotional healing, and personal growth. For individuals with bipolar disorder, engaging in creative endeavors can be empowering and therapeutic, complementing traditional treatment approaches. This essay explores the use of art, music, and other creative therapies in the context of bipolar disorder, shedding light on their potential benefits, considerations, and integration into a comprehensive treatment plan.

Art Therapy:

Art therapy utilizes various art forms, such as painting, drawing, sculpture, or collage, to facilitate self, expression and emotional healing. It provides a non, verbal and non, judgmental means of communication, allowing individuals to explore and process their thoughts, feelings, and experiences. Engaging in art therapy can enhance self, awareness, promote emotional regulation, and provide a sense of empowerment for individuals with bipolar disorder.

Music Therapy:

Music therapy involves the use of music, such as listening, playing instruments, or singing, to support emotional, cognitive, and social well, being. It harnesses the power of music to facilitate self, expression, reduce stress, and enhance mood regulation. Engaging in music therapy can help individuals with bipolar disorder manage their emotions, improve self, esteem, and develop healthy coping mechanisms.

Dance/Movement Therapy:

Dance/movement therapy combines movement, creative expression, and therapeutic principles to promote emotional integration and well, being.

It provides a safe space for individuals with bipolar disorder to explore their bodies, express emotions, and enhance self, awareness. Engaging in dance/movement therapy can improve body image, reduce stress, and support emotional regulation.

Writing/Journaling:

Writing and journaling provide an outlet for self, reflection, emotional processing, and personal growth. It allows individuals with bipolar disorder to articulate their thoughts, feelings, and experiences, facilitating a deeper understanding of themselves. Writing can serve as a form of self, care, helping individuals navigate mood fluctuations, manage stress, and foster resilience.

Drama/Therapeutic Theater:

Drama and therapeutic theater utilize improvisation, role, playing, and storytelling to promote self, expression, empathy, and personal growth. Engaging in these activities can help individuals with bipolar disorder explore different perspectives, develop emotional resilience, and enhance interpersonal skills. Drama and therapeutic theater provide a safe space for creative exploration and self, discovery.

Benefits of Creative Therapies for Bipolar Disorder:

Emotional Expression and Regulation: Creative therapies provide a non, verbal outlet for individuals with bipolar disorder to express and regulate their emotions. They offer alternative channels for processing intense feelings, reducing emotional distress, and promoting emotional balance.

Stress Reduction: Engaging in creative activities can reduce stress and anxiety, which are common triggers for mood episodes in bipolar disorder. Creative therapies provide a constructive and enjoyable means of relaxation and self, soothing.

Self, Exploration and Self, Awareness: Creative therapies encourage self, reflection and introspection, fostering a deeper understanding of one's thoughts, feelings, and triggers. They can facilitate self, acceptance, personal growth, and the development of healthy coping mechanisms.

Sense of Control and Empowerment: Engaging in creative endeavors empowers individuals with bipolar disorder by allowing them to take control of their artistic process. It provides a sense of agency, mastery, and accomplishment.

Social Connection and Support: Participating in group, based creative therapies promotes social interaction, a sense of belonging, and mutual support. It reduces feelings of isolation and fosters a supportive community for individuals with bipolar disorder.

Chapter Twenty-Seven

Bipolar Disorder and Technology

Harnessing the Digital Realm: Exploring Bipolar Disorder and Technology

Technology has become an integral part of our daily lives, shaping how we communicate, work, and engage with the world. For individuals with bipolar disorder, technology offers a range of opportunities, from support tools to potential triggers. This essay explores the relationship between bipolar disorder and technology, delving into the potential benefits, considerations, and responsible usage of technology in managing the condition.

Mental Health Apps and Online Resources:

Technology has given rise to a multitude of mental health apps and online resources designed to support individuals with bipolar disorder. These apps offer features such as mood tracking, medication reminders, coping strategies, and access to support networks. While these tools can enhance self, awareness and self, management, it is important to select reputable and evidence, based apps and consult healthcare professionals for guidance.

Teletherapy and Online Support Groups:

Teletherapy, also known as online therapy or e, counseling, allows individuals with bipolar disorder to access mental health support from the comfort of their own homes. Online support groups provide a platform for individuals to connect, share experiences, and offer mutual support. Teletherapy and online support groups can enhance accessibility and reduce barriers to mental health care.

Education and Information:

The internet provides a vast array of educational resources and information about bipolar disorder. Online platforms, websites, and forums offer a wealth of knowledge about the condition, treatment options, and coping strategies. However, it is essential to critically evaluate sources and seek information from reputable websites and healthcare professionals to ensure accuracy and reliability.

Self, Care and Well, being:

Technology can support self, care and well, being for individuals with bipolar disorder. Meditation and mindfulness apps provide guided practices that promote relaxation and emotional regulation. Fitness apps and wearable devices can assist in tracking physical activity and sleep patterns, both of which are essential for mood stability. Digital journaling and creative apps offer platforms for self, expression and emotional processing.

Remote Monitoring and Digital Health Tools:

Remote monitoring and digital health tools allow healthcare providers to remotely monitor individuals with bipolar disorder, track symptoms, and adjust treatment plans accordingly. These tools can enhance communication between patients and healthcare professionals, providing real, time insights and promoting proactive management of the condition.

Potential Triggers and Risks:

While technology offers many benefits, it is important to be aware of potential triggers and risks for individuals with bipolar disorder. Excessive screen time and social media use can contribute to feelings of isolation, comparison, and instability. The constant availability of information and notifications can exacerbate stress and disrupt sleep patterns. Being mindful of personal boundaries, setting screen, time limits, and engaging in digital detoxes can help mitigate these risks.

Responsible Digital Engagement:

Responsible digital engagement involves using technology in a mindful and balanced manner. Setting boundaries, such as designated screen, free time, can help individuals with bipolar disorder maintain stability and protect their mental well, being. Cultivating healthy online habits, such as connecting with positive communities and avoiding triggering content, can promote a supportive digital environment.

Cybersecurity and Privacy:

Individuals with bipolar disorder should prioritize cybersecurity and privacy when using technology. Protecting personal information, using secure networks, and being cautious about sharing sensitive details online are essential. Trusting reputable mental health apps and ensuring they prioritize user privacy and data security is crucial.

Seeking Professional Guidance:

While technology can be a valuable tool in managing bipolar disorder, it should not replace professional guidance and treatment. It is important to consult with healthcare professionals to determine the most appropriate use of technology in an individual's treatment plan. Healthcare professionals can provide tailored recommendations, monitor progress, and offer guidance on responsible technology usage.

Smartphone apps and online tools for mood tracking

Mood in Your Pocket: Exploring Smartphone Apps and Online Tools for Mood Tracking in Bipolar Disorders

In the era of digital advancements, smartphones have become an integral part of our lives, providing a wealth of resources at our fingertips. For individuals with bipolar disorder, smartphone apps and online tools offer a convenient and accessible way to track mood fluctuations, gain insights into their mental health, and support self, management. This essay explores the role of smartphone apps and online tools in mood tracking for individuals with bipolar disorder, highlighting their benefits, considerations, and potential impact on managing the condition.

Mood Tracking Apps:

Mood tracking apps provide a user, friendly platform for individuals to record and monitor their moods, emotions, and other relevant factors. These apps often employ visual interfaces, customizable features, and reminders to facilitate consistent mood tracking. By documenting daily experiences, individuals with bipolar disorder can gain a deeper understanding of their emotional patterns and identify triggers or warning signs of mood episodes.

Symptom Monitoring:

In addition to mood tracking, smartphone apps can help monitor other symptoms associated with bipolar disorder, such as sleep patterns, energy levels, medication adherence, and treatment responses. By tracking these variables over time, individuals can identify patterns and share valuable data with healthcare professionals during appointments, aiding in treatment decisions and adjustments.

Insights and Patterns:

Smartphone apps and online tools often provide visual representations, charts, and summaries of mood data, allowing users to identify trends, patterns, and correlations between mood fluctuations and various factors. This feature can help individuals recognize associations between mood episodes and specific triggers, such as sleep disturbances, stressful events, or changes in medication regimens. By gaining insights into these patterns, individuals can make informed decisions about self, care and seek professional support when necessary.

Medication Reminders and Management:

Many mood tracking apps offer features to set medication reminders and track medication adherence. These reminders can be particularly useful for individuals with bipolar disorder who require regular medication intake for mood stabilization. Maintaining a consistent medication routine is vital in managing bipolar symptoms, and these apps can help individuals stay on track and improve treatment outcomes.

Communication with Healthcare Providers:

Some mood tracking apps facilitate communication and data sharing between individuals and their healthcare providers. s can export or email their mood data, symptom records, and notes to their healthcare team, promoting collaborative decision, making and more productive appointments. This feature enhances the therapeutic alliance and ensures that treatment plans are tailored to individual needs.

Self, Awareness and Empowerment:

Engaging with mood tracking apps fosters self, awareness and empowers individuals to actively participate in their mental health management. Regularly monitoring moods and symptoms helps individuals recognize their emotional patterns, identify potential triggers, and make informed choices about self, care strategies. This heightened self, awareness can contribute to a greater sense of control, improved coping skills, and enhanced well, being.

Considerations for Accuracy and Reliability:

While mood tracking apps can be beneficial, it is important to consider their accuracy and reliability. Some apps rely solely on user input, which may be subjective and prone to biases. Others incorporate data from wearable devices, such as smartwatches, to capture physiological indicators like heart rate or sleep quality. It is crucial to choose reputable and evidence, based apps, and consult with healthcare professionals for recommendations.

Personalization and Privacy:

Every individual with bipolar disorder experiences unique symptoms and triggers. Therefore, it is essential to select mood tracking apps that offer customization options to align with specific needs. Additionally, privacy and data security should be prioritized. Selecting apps that adhere to data protection protocols and allow users to control their information's visibility and sharing is vital to maintaining confidentiality and privacy.

Teletherapy and remote mental health services

Bridging the Distance: Exploring Teletherapy and Remote Mental Health Services for Bipolar Disorders

In today's digital age, technology has revolutionized the way we access healthcare services, including mental health support. Teletherapy and remote mental health services offer individuals with bipolar disorder convenient and accessible options for receiving therapy, counseling, and support from the comfort of their own homes. This essay explores the role of teletherapy and remote mental health services in managing bipolar disorders, highlighting their benefits, considerations, and potential impact on treatment outcomes.

Accessible Mental Health Support:

Teletherapy and remote mental health services break down geographical barriers, providing individuals with bipolar disorder access to mental health professionals regardless of their location. This is particularly beneficial for individuals residing in rural areas or areas with limited mental health resources. Teletherapy ensures that individuals can connect with qualified professionals and receive timely support without the need for physical travel.

Convenience and Flexibility:

Teletherapy eliminates the need for in, person appointments, offering convenience and flexibility to individuals with bipolar disorder. Remote sessions can be scheduled at mutually convenient times, allowing individuals to integrate therapy into their daily routines more seamlessly. This flexibility is especially valuable for those managing work, family responsibilities, or physical health limitations.

Enhanced Comfort and Privacy:

For individuals with bipolar disorder, privacy and comfort are crucial factors in seeking mental health support. Teletherapy provides a safe and private environment for therapy sessions, reducing the potential stigma associated with in, person visits to a mental health clinic. This sense of privacy can encourage individuals to openly share their experiences, emotions, and concerns, leading to more effective therapeutic outcomes.

Continuity of Care:

Bipolar disorder often requires ongoing, consistent mental health support. Teletherapy ensures continuity of care, especially during times when in, person sessions may be challenging, such as during travel or unexpected disruptions. This continuity helps maintain treatment progress and supports the development of a strong therapeutic relationship between the individual and their mental health professional.

Tailored Treatment Options:

Teletherapy offers a wide range of therapeutic approaches tailored to the unique needs of individuals with bipolar disorder. Cognitive, behavioral therapy (CBT), dialectical behavior therapy (DBT), and psychoeducation can be effectively delivered through teletherapy platforms. Additionally, remote mental health services provide specialized treatment options, such as support groups or programs specifically designed for bipolar disorder management.

Remote Monitoring and Self, Management:

Teletherapy platforms often include features for remote monitoring and self, management of bipolar disorder symptoms. Some platforms offer mood tracking tools, activity monitoring, and reminders for medication adherence. These features enable individuals to actively participate in their treatment, track their progress, and make informed decisions about self, care strategies between therapy sessions.

Support During Crisis and Relapse Prevention:

Bipolar disorder is characterized by recurrent episodes of depression and mania, with the potential for crisis situations. Teletherapy provides a lifeline during such times, offering immediate support and intervention. It allows individuals to reach out to their mental health professionals promptly, facilitating crisis management and relapse prevention strategies.

Considerations and Limitations:

Despite the benefits, teletherapy and remote mental health services have certain considerations and limitations. Reliable internet connectivity and access to appropriate technology are prerequisites for effective teletherapy. Additionally, individuals with severe symptoms, acute crisis situations, or complex mental health needs may require in, person interventions and should consult with healthcare professionals to determine the most suitable treatment approach.

Building Rapport and Therapeutic Alliance:

Establishing a strong therapeutic alliance is essential for successful treatment outcomes. Teletherapy relies on effective communication through video or audio platforms, and building rapport may require additional effort compared to in, person sessions. Mental health professionals practicing teletherapy employ techniques to facilitate connection and ensure that individuals feel heard, understood, and supported.

Virtual support groups and social networks

Connected in Community: Exploring Virtual Support Groups and Social Networks for Bipolar Disorders

Living with bipolar disorder can be challenging, but finding a supportive community can make a significant difference in managing the condition. Virtual support groups and social networks offer individuals with bipolar disorder the opportunity to connect with others who share similar experiences, gain valuable insights, and receive emotional support. This essay explores the role of virtual support groups and social networks in the context of bipolar disorders, highlighting their benefits, considerations, and potential impact on well, being.

Access to Peer Support:

Virtual support groups and social networks provide individuals with bipolar disorder access to a supportive community of peers who understand the challenges and nuances of living with the condition. Connecting with others who have firsthand experience fosters empathy, validation, and a sense of belonging. Peer support can help reduce feelings of isolation, provide encouragement, and offer practical advice based on shared experiences.

Sharing Knowledge and Information:

Virtual support groups and social networks serve as platforms for sharing knowledge and information related to bipolar disorder. Individuals can exchange insights on coping strategies, medication management, therapy techniques, and self, care practices. These communities facilitate the dissemination of accurate, up, to, date information and empower individuals to become informed advocates for their own well, being.

Emotional Validation and Empathy:

Bipolar disorder is often accompanied by emotional ups and downs, and navigating these fluctuations can be overwhelming. Virtual support groups and social networks offer a space for individuals to express their emotions, share their triumphs and challenges, and receive validation and empathy from others who can relate. This emotional support can alleviate feelings of loneliness, foster a sense of understanding, and enhance emotional well, being.

Anonymous and Non, Judgmental Environment:

Virtual support groups and social networks provide an anonymous and non, judgmental environment for individuals to openly discuss their experiences with bipolar disorder. Anonymity allows individuals to feel more comfortable sharing personal stories, concerns, and vulnerabilities without fear of stigma or discrimination. This environment promotes open dialogue, self, expression, and mutual support.

24/7 Availability and Flexibility:

One of the advantages of virtual support groups and social networks is their accessibility at any time, providing individuals with bipolar disorder the flexibility to engage and participate according to their needs and schedules. This around, the, clock availability ensures that individuals can access support, guidance, and encouragement whenever they require it, fostering a continuous support system.

Diverse Perspectives and Global Reach:

Virtual support groups and social networks have a global reach, connecting individuals from diverse backgrounds and cultures. This diversity brings a richness of perspectives and experiences, broadening individuals' understanding of bipolar disorder and its impact. Engaging with a global community allows for the exchange of ideas, cultural insights, and the opportunity to learn from a wide range of perspectives.

Parent and Family Support:

Bipolar disorder not only affects individuals living with the condition but also has an impact on their family members and loved ones. Virtual support groups and social networks offer dedicated spaces for parents and families of individuals with bipolar disorder to seek support, share experiences, and learn coping strategies. These groups provide a network of understanding and guidance for caregivers, promoting their well, being as well.

Professional Guidance and Moderation:

Many virtual support groups and social networks have moderators or mental health professionals who provide guidance, facilitate discussions, and ensure a safe and supportive environment. Their presence helps maintain respectful communication, offers expert insights, and directs individuals to appropriate resources when needed. Professional moderation ensures that accurate information is shared and harmful content is minimized.

Chapter Twenty-Eight

Cultural Perspectives on Bipolar Disorder

Shaping Understanding: Cultural Perspectives on Bipolar Disorder

Bipolar disorder is a complex mental health condition that affects individuals worldwide. Cultural perspectives play a significant role in shaping the understanding, interpretation, and management of bipolar disorder within different communities. This essay explores the diverse cultural perspectives on bipolar disorder, highlighting the ways in which culture influences its perception, treatment, seeking behavior, and stigma associated with the condition.

Cultural Variations in Symptom Expression:

Bipolar disorder manifests differently across cultures, with variations in symptom expression and interpretation. In some cultures, manic or hypomanic episodes may be viewed as a sign of heightened creativity or spiritual experiences, while depressive episodes may be attributed to personal weaknesses or moral failings. Understanding cultural variations in symptom expression is crucial for accurate diagnosis and culturally sensitive treatment approaches.

Traditional Healing Practices:

Many cultures have traditional healing practices that offer alternative approaches to managing bipolar disorder. These practices may involve rituals, herbal remedies, or spiritual interventions. Traditional healers or shamans may play a significant role in the treatment process, addressing the physical, psychological, and spiritual aspects of the condition. It is essential to acknowledge and respect the cultural beliefs and practices that individuals may incorporate into their treatment journey.

Influence of Religion and Spirituality:

Religion and spirituality often intersect with cultural perspectives on bipolar disorder. Some religious beliefs may attribute the condition to spiritual possession or divine punishment. Conversely, spiritual practices and religious communities can provide support, solace, and a sense of purpose for individuals with bipolar disorder. Understanding the role of religion and spirituality in the lives of individuals with bipolar disorder is crucial for providing culturally sensitive care.

Help, Seeking Behavior:

Cultural beliefs and attitudes towards mental health influence help, seeking behavior. In some cultures, seeking professional help for mental health concerns is stigmatized or discouraged due to fear of judgment or social consequences. Instead, individuals may rely on informal support networks, such as family, friends, or community leaders. Recognizing cultural barriers to help, seeking and promoting mental health awareness within specific cultural contexts is essential.

Stigma and Discrimination:

Stigma associated with bipolar disorder varies across cultures and can have profound impacts on individuals' lives. Cultural perceptions that equate mental illness with weakness or shame contribute to the social stigma surrounding bipolar disorder. Stigmatization can lead to discrimination, isolation, and hinder individuals from accessing appropriate care. Addressing stigma requires community education, advocacy, and fostering open conversations about mental health.

Cultural Competence in Treatment:

Cultural competence in mental health care involves understanding and respecting cultural perspectives, beliefs, and practices. Mental health professionals should strive to develop cultural competence by educating themselves about the cultural contexts in which individuals with bipolar disorder live. This includes considering cultural interpretations of symptoms, incorporating culturally appropriate interventions, and fostering culturally sensitive therapeutic relationships.

Family and Community Support:

In many cultures, the family unit plays a vital role in supporting individuals with bipolar disorder. Families often provide emotional, financial, and practical support, and involvement in treatment decisions. Community support networks, such as support groups or cultural associations, can also offer invaluable support and understanding. Recognizing the importance of family and community involvement is crucial for effective treatment planning and ongoing support.

Language and Communication:

Cultural perspectives on bipolar disorder are communicated through language, which may vary in the ways it conceptualizes mental health. The use of culturally sensitive language and effective communication strategies is essential in building trust, understanding, and engagement with individuals from diverse cultural backgrounds. Mental health professionals should strive to bridge language barriers and promote effective communication for accurate assessment and treatment.

Cross

,

cultural variations in diagnosis and treatment

Cultural Kaleidoscope: Exploring Cross, Cultural Variations in the Diagnosis and Treatment of Bipolar Disorder

Bipolar disorder is a complex mental health condition that manifests differently across cultures. The diagnosis and treatment of bipolar disorder are influenced by cultural perspectives, beliefs, and healthcare systems. This essay explores the cross, cultural variations in the diagnosis and treatment of bipolar disorder, shedding light on the diverse approaches, challenges, and considerations within different cultural contexts.

Diagnostic Variations:

Diagnostic criteria for bipolar disorder, such as the DSM, 5 (Diagnostic and Statistical Manual of Mental Disorders), provide a standardized framework. However, cultural variations in symptom presentation and interpretations may influence the diagnosis. Cultural nuances in understanding and expressing emotions, distress, and mood episodes can impact the recognition and labeling of bipolar symptoms. Cultural competence in diagnosis requires sensitivity to these variations.

Cultural Idioms of Distress:

Cultures often have unique idioms of distress, or culturally specific ways of expressing psychological distress. These idioms may encompass somatic complaints, spiritual experiences, or cultural syndromes that resemble bipolar symptoms. Mental health professionals need to be aware of these cultural expressions to accurately assess and diagnose bipolar disorder. Collaboration with cultural consultants or interpreters may be necessary for accurate understanding.

Traditional Healing Practices:

Traditional healing practices rooted in cultural beliefs and traditions can influence the treatment of bipolar disorder. Indigenous healing systems, such as Ayurveda, Traditional Chinese Medicine, or Native American healing practices, may incorporate herbal remedies, acupuncture, or spiritual rituals. Integrating traditional healing practices with evidence, based treatments can be crucial for individuals who value cultural traditions and seek holistic care.

Access to Mental Health Services:

Cross, cultural variations in access to mental health services significantly impact diagnosis and treatment. Disparities in healthcare infrastructure, economic resources, and geographical location affect the availability and affordability of mental health services. Limited access can lead to delayed diagnosis, inadequate treatment, and increased reliance on informal support systems. Addressing these disparities is essential to ensure equitable mental healthcare for all cultural groups.

Stigma and Help, Seeking:

Stigma associated with mental illness varies across cultures and profoundly influences help, seeking behavior. Cultural beliefs, values, and norms may perpetuate stigmatization, leading individuals to hide their symptoms or avoid seeking professional help. The perception of mental illness as a source of shame or personal failure can deter individuals from accessing appropriate diagnosis and treatment. Promoting mental health awareness and combating stigma are crucial for early intervention and improved outcomes.

Cultural Beliefs about Medication:

Cultural beliefs about medication can influence treatment adherence and acceptance. Some cultural groups may have reservations about psychiatric medications due to concerns about side effects, dependency, or mistrust of Western medicine. Culturally sensitive education and communication are necessary to address misconceptions, provide information about treatment options, and establish collaborative decision, making regarding medication use.

Therapeutic Relationships and Cultural Competence:

Cultural competence in the therapeutic relationship is essential for effective treatment. Mental health professionals need to understand the cultural contexts, values, and communication styles of the individuals they serve. Developing cultural competence involves active listening, respect for diverse perspectives, and adapting therapeutic approaches to align with cultural beliefs and preferences. Collaborating with cultural consultants or seeking cultural training can enhance cultural competence.

Family and Community Involvement:

Family and community play crucial roles in the treatment of bipolar disorder across cultures. In some cultures, family members are actively involved in treatment decisions, providing support and participating in therapy sessions. Cultural beliefs about the interconnectedness of family and mental health may influence treatment approaches, requiring mental health professionals to collaborate with families and recognize their valuable contributions.

Addressing cultural stigma and barriers to care

Breaking Barriers: Addressing Cultural Stigma and Barriers to Care in Bipolar Disorders

Cultural stigma surrounding mental health conditions, including bipolar disorder, continues to pose significant barriers to diagnosis, treatment, and support. Understanding and addressing cultural stigma is crucial to ensure individuals with bipolar disorder receive timely and appropriate care. This essay explores the cultural stigma and barriers to care experienced by individuals with bipolar disorder, highlighting strategies to overcome these challenges and promote mental health well, being within diverse cultural contexts.

Cultural Perspectives on Mental Health:

Cultural perspectives shape attitudes, beliefs, and understanding of mental health conditions. In some cultures, mental illness is stigmatized, leading to negative stereotypes, discrimination, and social exclusion. Cultural norms and values may view mental health challenges as personal weaknesses or spiritual issues, contributing to the reluctance to seek professional help. Sensitivity to cultural perspectives is essential to challenge and address the associated stigma.

Language and Cultural Competence:

Effective communication plays a vital role in combating stigma and addressing barriers to care. Mental health professionals should strive to bridge language and cultural gaps, using culturally sensitive language and communication styles. Culturally competent care involves understanding cultural norms, beliefs, and idioms of distress related to bipolar disorder. Training programs and resources can help mental health professionals develop cultural competence in their practice.

Education and Awareness:

Education and awareness initiatives are key to challenging cultural stigma and increasing mental health literacy within communities. By providing accurate information about bipolar disorder, its symptoms, and available treatments, education initiatives can dispel myths and misconceptions. Awareness campaigns should be tailored to specific cultural contexts, utilizing culturally relevant strategies and involving community leaders, religious organizations, and influential figures.

Community Engagement and Support:

Engaging community leaders and organizations is essential for addressing cultural stigma and promoting mental health support. Collaborating with community groups can facilitate open discussions, normalize conversations about mental health, and develop culturally appropriate support networks. Culturally sensitive support groups and initiatives that empower individuals with bipolar disorder can help reduce isolation and foster a sense of belonging.

Family Involvement and Psychoeducation:

In many cultures, family plays a central role in decision, making and support for individuals with bipolar disorder. Engaging families through psychoeducation initiatives provides a platform for understanding the condition, dispelling myths, and promoting acceptance. Educating families about bipolar disorder symptoms, treatment options, and available resources empowers them to provide effective support and reduces the stigma within family structures.

Integration of Traditional Healing Practices:

Acknowledging and integrating traditional healing practices into the treatment of bipolar disorder can help address cultural stigma and enhance

access to care. Collaborating with traditional healers, incorporating culturally appropriate therapies, or integrating holistic approaches can bridge the gap between biomedical and traditional healing systems. Respect for cultural beliefs and values promotes a comprehensive and inclusive approach to treatment.

Culturally Competent Mental Health Services:

Mental health services should be culturally competent, providing a safe and inclusive environment for individuals seeking care. Culturally competent services recognize and respect cultural beliefs, practices, and customs. This includes ensuring a diverse workforce, providing interpreters when necessary, and addressing potential cultural biases within the mental health system. Building trust through culturally competent care can encourage individuals to seek help without fear of discrimination.

Collaboration and Partnerships:

Collaboration between mental health professionals, community leaders, advocacy groups, and policymakers is crucial in addressing cultural stigma and barriers to care. Partnerships can lead to the development of culturally sensitive policies, improved access to mental health services, and increased resources for mental health promotion within diverse communities. By working together, stakeholders can create a comprehensive framework for addressing cultural stigma and promoting mental health equity.

Incorporating cultural sensitivity in mental health care

Embracing Diversity: Incorporating Cultural Sensitivity in Bipolar Disorder Mental Health Care

Cultural sensitivity is a fundamental aspect of providing effective and equitable mental health care for individuals with bipolar disorder. Recognizing and addressing the diverse cultural backgrounds, beliefs, and practices of individuals is crucial for fostering trust, reducing disparities, and ensuring positive treatment outcomes. This essay explores the importance of cultural sensitivity in mental health care for bipolar disorder, highlighting strategies and considerations to promote culturally competent practices.

Understanding Cultural Contexts:

Cultural sensitivity begins with understanding the unique cultural contexts in which individuals with bipolar disorder live. Mental health professionals should familiarize themselves with the cultural norms, values, beliefs, and idioms of distress associated with bipolar disorder within diverse communities. Recognizing the influence of cultural factors on symptom expression, help, seeking behaviors, and treatment preferences is essential for providing personalized and effective care.

Culturally Competent Assessment:

Conducting culturally competent assessments involves using culturally sensitive and relevant tools to evaluate the symptoms and impact of bipolar disorder. This may include adapting assessment measures to consider cultural expressions of distress, incorporating cultural idioms, and acknowledging the influence of cultural beliefs on help, seeking behaviors. By understanding the cultural context, mental health professionals can develop accurate diagnoses and treatment plans.

Effective Communication:

Effective communication is at the heart of culturally sensitive mental health care. Mental health professionals should be mindful of language barriers, employing interpreters or translators when necessary. Using culturally appropriate language and communication styles, such as active listening and empathy, fosters trust and understanding. Open dialogue allows individuals to express their experiences, concerns, and beliefs, contributing to more personalized and effective care.

Incorporating Cultural Beliefs and Practices:

Cultural sensitivity involves recognizing and respecting cultural beliefs and practices related to bipolar disorder. Mental health professionals should be open to integrating culturally relevant approaches into treatment plans, collaborating with individuals and their families. This may include incorporating traditional healing practices, religious or spiritual rituals, or cultural interventions that align with the individual's beliefs and preferences.

Addressing Stigma and Reducing Bias:

Cultural sensitivity requires actively addressing and challenging the stigma associated with bipolar disorder within specific cultural contexts. Mental health professionals should promote education, raise awareness, and challenge misconceptions through culturally tailored anti, stigma campaigns. Additionally, clinicians must examine their own biases and cultural assumptions to ensure they provide non, judgmental and unbiased care.

Collaborative Decision, Making:

Culturally sensitive care involves adopting a collaborative approach to decision, making. Mental health professionals should engage individuals with bipolar disorder in the treatment process, valuing their input, and incorporating their cultural preferences. Encouraging individuals to actively participate in decision, making empowers them, fosters a sense of ownership, and enhances treatment adherence and satisfaction.

Cultural Competence Training:

Continual professional development through cultural competence training is essential for mental health professionals. Training programs can provide education on cultural diversity, cultural humility, and the intersectionality of identity. These initiatives promote self, reflection, challenge biases, and enhance awareness of cultural factors that influence the experience of bipolar disorder. Culturally competent mental health professionals can better understand and address the specific needs of individuals from diverse backgrounds.

Diverse Workforce and Cultural Representation:

Ensuring a diverse workforce within the mental health field is important for providing culturally sensitive care. Encouraging recruitment and training of mental health professionals from diverse backgrounds can enhance cultural representation and foster trust among individuals seeking care. By having mental health professionals who share similar cultural backgrounds or have undergone cultural competency training, individuals with bipolar disorder can feel understood and supported.

Chapter Twenty-Nine

Bipolar Disorder and LGBTQ+ Communities

Navigating Dual Identities: Bipolar Disorder and the LGBTQ+ Communities

Bipolar disorder affects individuals across diverse communities, including the lesbian, gay, bisexual, transgender, and queer (LGBTQ+) population. Understanding the intersectionality of bipolar disorder and LGBTQ+ identities is crucial for providing effective mental health care. This essay explores the unique experiences, challenges, and considerations related to bipolar disorder within the LGBTQ+ communities, highlighting the importance of culturally sensitive and inclusive approaches to treatment.

Intersectionality and Minority Stress:

LGBTQ+ individuals often face unique stressors and challenges, such as societal discrimination, stigma, and lack of acceptance. These experiences, known as minority stress, can contribute to higher rates of mental health conditions, including bipolar disorder. Recognizing the intersectionality of LGBTQ+ identities and bipolar disorder allows mental health professionals to provide comprehensive care that addresses the specific needs and experiences of this population.

Coming Out and Bipolar Disorder:

The process of coming out can be emotionally complex for individuals with bipolar disorder. The added stress and anxiety of revealing one's sexual orientation or gender identity can trigger mood episodes or exacerbate existing symptoms. Mental health professionals should provide a supportive environment and address the unique challenges faced by LGBTQ+ individuals with bipolar disorder during the coming out process.

Gender Dysphoria and Mood Disorders:

Gender dysphoria, the distress caused by a mismatch between one's assigned sex at birth and their gender identity, can impact the mental health of transgender and gender, diverse individuals. The experience of gender dysphoria, coupled with bipolar disorder, may increase the risk of mood disorders and complicate treatment. Mental health professionals should adopt an inclusive and affirming approach when working with transgender and gender, diverse individuals with bipolar disorder.

Healthcare Disparities and Access to Care:

LGBTQ+ individuals often encounter healthcare disparities, including barriers to accessing mental health care. Discrimination, lack of cultural competence, and fears of mistreatment or rejection can prevent LGBTQ+ individuals with bipolar disorder from seeking help. Mental health professionals must address these disparities by providing LGBTQ+ inclusive and affirming environments, training staff in cultural competency, and actively engaging with LGBTQ+ organizations to increase accessibility to care.

Dual Minority Identity:

The intersection of bipolar disorder and LGBTQ+ identities presents unique challenges for individuals navigating dual minority identities. Bipolar disorder may impact an individual's self, acceptance, mental health, and experiences within the LGBTQ+ community. Mental health professionals should address the specific needs and concerns related to both identities, providing support that recognizes and validates the individual's experiences.

Acceptance and Social Support:

Acceptance within the LGBTQ+ community is crucial for the well, being of individuals with bipolar disorder. A supportive and affirming social network can act as a protective factor, reducing stigma, and promoting mental health resilience. Mental health professionals should encourage individuals to seek out LGBTQ+, inclusive support groups, organizations, and online communities that offer understanding, validation, and a sense of belonging.

Cultural Competence and LGBTQ+ Affirming Care:

Cultural competence in mental health care involves understanding and addressing the unique experiences and needs of LGBTQ+ individuals with bipolar disorder. Mental health professionals should educate themselves on LGBTQ+ terminology, the impact of societal prejudice, and the specific mental health concerns faced by this population. By providing LGBTQ+ affirming care, mental health professionals can foster trust, encourage help, seeking, and enhance treatment outcomes.

Transition, Related Care and Medication Interactions:

For transgender individuals with bipolar disorder, the interaction between bipolar medication and hormone therapy should be carefully considered. Mental health professionals should collaborate with healthcare providers experienced in transgender health to develop comprehensive treatment plans that address both the mental health needs and the unique medical considerations of transgender individuals.

Prevalence and unique challenges faced by LGBTQ+ individuals

Embracing Diversity: Prevalence and Unique Challenges Faced by LGBTQ+ Individuals with Bipolar Disorder

LGBTQ+ individuals experience unique challenges related to their sexual orientation, gender identity, and mental health. When combined with bipolar disorder, these challenges can further impact well, being and quality of life. This essay explores the prevalence of bipolar disorder within the LGBTQ+ community and highlights the unique challenges faced by LGBTQ+ individuals in relation to their mental health, emphasizing the importance of inclusive and culturally sensitive approaches to care.

Prevalence of Bipolar Disorder:

Research indicates that LGBTQ+ individuals may have higher rates of mental health conditions, including bipolar disorder, compared to the general population. Minority stress, discrimination, and social disparities contribute to increased vulnerability to mood disorders. Understanding the prevalence of bipolar disorder within the LGBTQ+ community is vital for providing appropriate support and tailored interventions.

Intersectionality and Multiple Identities:

The experiences of LGBTQ+ individuals are multifaceted, encompassing diverse sexual orientations, gender identities, racial backgrounds, and socioeconomic statuses. The intersectionality of these identities influences mental health outcomes and the experience of bipolar disorder. Mental health professionals should acknowledge and address the complex interplay of these identities to provide inclusive and affirming care.

Discrimination, Stigma, and Minority Stress:

LGBTQ+ individuals often face discrimination, stigma, and prejudice, which can significantly impact mental health. The cumulative effect of minority stress, resulting from societal rejection and marginalization, increases the risk of mood disorders and exacerbates symptoms of bipolar disorder. Culturally sensitive care should aim to mitigate the effects of discrimination, provide validation, and create a safe and accepting environment for LGBTQ+ individuals.

Coming Out and Bipolar Disorder:

The process of coming out can be uniquely challenging for individuals with bipolar disorder. The emotional upheaval and additional stress of disclosing one's sexual orientation or gender identity may trigger mood episodes or affect treatment adherence. Mental health professionals should provide support and guidance during the coming out process, addressing the specific needs and concerns of LGBTQ+ individuals with bipolar disorder.

Gender Dysphoria and Mood Disorders:

Transgender and gender, diverse individuals may experience gender dysphoria, which involves distress related to a misalignment between one's gender identity and assigned sex at birth. The experience of gender dysphoria, combined with bipolar disorder, can contribute to additional mental health challenges. Mental health professionals should adopt an inclusive and gender, affirming approach to address the unique needs and concerns of transgender and gender, diverse individuals with bipolar disorder.

Barriers to Care:

LGBTQ+ individuals face various barriers to accessing mental health care, including healthcare disparities, lack of cultural competence, and fear of discrimination or judgment. These barriers may hinder help, seeking behaviors and delay treatment. Culturally sensitive mental health services should actively work to reduce barriers by providing LGBTQ+ inclusive and affirming environments, training staff in LGBTQ+ competency, and increasing accessibility to care for all individuals.

Social Support and Acceptance:

Social support and acceptance play a vital role in the mental health and well, being of LGBTQ+ individuals with bipolar disorder. Building affirming social networks, including friends, family, and LGBTQ+ support groups, can help combat the effects of stigma and isolation. Mental health professionals should encourage the development of strong support systems and facilitate connections with LGBTQ+, friendly resources and organizations.

Mental Health Disparities:

LGBTQ+ individuals face mental health disparities, including higher rates of depression, anxiety, and suicidal ideation. These disparities are exacerbated when bipolar disorder is present. Culturally sensitive care should address these disparities by promoting mental health awareness, offering LGBTQ+, specific resources and interventions, and providing tailored support for LGBTQ+ individuals with bipolar disorder.

Affirming mental health care for LGBTQ+ people

Embracing Authenticity: Affirming Mental Health Care for LGBTQ+ Individuals with Bipolar Disorder

Affirming mental health care is essential for promoting the well, being of LGBTQ+ individuals with bipolar disorder. Recognizing and addressing the unique needs and challenges faced by this community can contribute to positive treatment outcomes and enhanced quality of life. This essay explores the importance of affirming mental health care for LGBTQ+ individuals with bipolar disorder, highlighting strategies and considerations for providing inclusive and culturally sensitive support.

Culturally Competent Approach:

Culturally competent care requires mental health professionals to have knowledge and understanding of LGBTQ+ identities, experiences, and mental health disparities. Familiarity with LGBTQ+ terminology, gender identities, and sexual orientations promotes a safe and inclusive environment for individuals with bipolar disorder. Mental health professionals should continuously educate themselves on LGBTQ+ issues to deliver effective and affirming care.

Safe and Welcoming Environments:

Creating safe and welcoming environments is crucial for LGBTQ+ individuals with bipolar disorder to feel comfortable and supported in seeking mental health care. This includes ensuring confidentiality, displaying LGBTQ+, inclusive signage and resources, and utilizing gender, affirming language and practices. The physical environment should be welcoming and free from discrimination, bias, or heteronormative assumptions.

LGBTQ+ Cultural Sensitivity:

Cultural sensitivity involves understanding and valuing the diverse experiences, norms, and values of LGBTQ+ individuals. Mental health professionals should demonstrate respect for gender identity, sexual orientation, and pronoun usage. Adopting a non, judgmental approach, actively listening, and avoiding assumptions fosters trust and enables individuals to share their unique experiences and concerns related to both bipolar disorder and LGBTQ+ identity.

Inclusive Assessment and Treatment Planning:

Assessment tools and treatment plans should be inclusive of LGBTQ+ experiences and address the specific needs of individuals with bipolar disorder. Culturally sensitive assessment should incorporate questions about sexual orientation, gender identity, and experiences of discrimination or minority stress. Treatment planning should consider the potential impact of gender dysphoria, coming out processes, or social support systems within the LGBTQ+ community.

Transgender and Non, Binary Affirming Care:

Transgender and non, binary individuals with bipolar disorder require gender, affirming care that recognizes and respects their gender identity. Mental health professionals should be knowledgeable about gender, affirming language, access to hormone therapy, and surgical interventions. Collaborating with transgender healthcare providers and providing psychoeducation about the interaction between bipolar medication and hormone therapy ensures comprehensive and holistic care.

Supporting Coming Out Processes:

Coming out is a significant milestone for many LGBTQ+ individuals and can be intertwined with their mental health journey. Mental health professionals should offer support, guidance, and resources during the coming out process. This may include exploring coping strategies, managing family dynamics, and addressing the emotional impact on bipolar symptoms. Affirming mental health care acknowledges the unique challenges and provides a safe space for individuals to navigate their identity.

LGBTQ+, Inclusive Support Networks:

Facilitating connections with LGBTQ+, inclusive support networks is vital for individuals with bipolar disorder. LGBTQ+ support groups, organizations, and online communities provide spaces for individuals to share experiences, find solidarity, and access relevant resources. Mental health professionals can provide information and referrals to LGBTQ+ community resources that offer specialized support and affirming spaces.

Collaboration with LGBTQ+ Community:

Collaborating with LGBTQ+ organizations and community leaders enhances the delivery of affirming mental health care. Mental health professionals can contribute their expertise, raise awareness about bipolar disorder within the LGBTQ+ community, and offer training on LGBTQ+ mental health. By working alongside LGBTQ+ community members, mental health professionals can better understand the unique challenges faced by this population and advocate for inclusive policies and services.

Support and resources for LGBTQ+ individuals with bipolar disorder

Embracing Resilience: Support and Resources for LGBTQ+ Individuals with Bipolar Disorder

LGBTQ+ individuals with bipolar disorder face unique challenges related to their sexual orientation, gender identity, and mental health. Access to appropriate support and resources is essential for promoting well, being and resilience within this population. This essay explores the importance of tailored support and available resources for LGBTQ+ individuals with bipolar disorder, highlighting the role of inclusive services in enhancing mental health outcomes and fostering a sense of belonging.

LGBTQ+, Affirming Mental Health Services:

LGBTQ+, affirming mental health services provide a safe and inclusive environment for individuals with bipolar disorder. These services are sensitive to the unique needs and experiences of LGBTQ+ individuals, fostering a sense of acceptance and understanding. Mental health professionals should undergo LGBTQ+ cultural competence training, ensuring that they can provide appropriate care and address specific concerns related to both bipolar disorder and LGBTQ+ identities.

LGBTQ+ Support Groups:

LGBTQ+ support groups offer a vital space for individuals with bipolar disorder to connect, share experiences, and find support within their community. These groups provide a sense of belonging and enable individuals to navigate the challenges associated with both their sexual orientation, gender identity, and bipolar disorder. Mental health professionals can refer individuals to LGBTQ+ support groups or facilitate the establishment of these groups within their practice or community.

Crisis Helplines and Hotlines:

Crisis helplines and hotlines specifically tailored to LGBTQ+ individuals provide immediate support for individuals in distress. These helplines are staffed with trained professionals who understand the unique challenges faced by LGBTQ+ individuals with bipolar disorder. They offer a confidential and understanding ear, provide information, and can assist in connecting individuals to appropriate resources and services.

LGBTQ+ Online Communities and Resources:

Online communities and resources play a crucial role in supporting LGBTQ+ individuals with bipolar disorder. Online platforms provide a space for individuals to share experiences, seek advice, and access information related to bipolar disorder and LGBTQ+ issues. Online resources can include articles, educational materials, mental health tools, and directories of LGBTQ+, affirming mental health professionals. These platforms foster a sense of community and can be particularly beneficial for individuals who may face barriers to in, person support.

LGBTQ+ Advocacy Organizations:

LGBTQ+ advocacy organizations work tirelessly to promote the rights, well, being, and mental health of LGBTQ+ individuals. These organizations provide valuable resources, educational campaigns, and advocacy efforts to address the specific challenges faced by LGBTQ+ individuals with bipolar disorder. Mental health professionals can collaborate with these organizations, support their initiatives, and refer individuals to their services and resources.

LGBTQ+, Friendly Healthcare Providers:

Accessing healthcare providers who are knowledgeable and affirming of LGBTQ+ identities is crucial for individuals with bipolar disorder. LGBTQ+, friendly healthcare providers understand the unique needs and concerns of LGBTQ+ individuals and provide a supportive and inclusive environment. Mental health professionals can connect individuals with bipolar disorder to LGBTQ+, friendly primary care physicians, endocrinologists, therapists, and psychiatrists, ensuring holistic and affirming care.

LGBTQ+ Cultural Competence Training for Mental Health Professionals:

Mental health professionals should undergo LGBTQ+ cultural competence training to better serve the needs of LGBTQ+ individuals with bipolar disorder. These training programs educate professionals about LGBTQ+ terminology, current research, cultural considerations, and specific mental health concerns. By developing cultural competence, mental health professionals can provide informed and sensitive care and contribute to reducing mental health disparities within the LGBTQ+ community.

LGBTQ+ Legal Support:

LGBTQ+ individuals may face legal challenges related to discrimination, employment, housing, or healthcare. Legal support services specifically focused on LGBTQ+ rights can provide assistance and guidance in navigating these legal complexities. Mental health professionals can inform individuals about their rights.

Chapter Thirty

Bipolar Disorder and Veterans

Navigating Battlefields Within: Bipolar Disorder and Veterans

Bipolar disorder is a complex mental health condition that can have profound effects on the lives of individuals, including veterans who have served in the military. Understanding the unique challenges faced by veterans with bipolar disorder is essential for providing effective support and care. This essay explores the intersection of bipolar disorder and the veteran experience, shedding light on the prevalence, risk factors, and specific considerations related to this population.

Prevalence and Risk Factors:

Veterans are at a higher risk of developing bipolar disorder compared to the general population. The unique stressors associated with military service, such as combat exposure, traumatic experiences, and multiple deployments, contribute to increased vulnerability. Additionally, the high prevalence of co, occurring mental health conditions, such as post, traumatic stress disorder (PTSD), substance abuse, and traumatic brain injury, further elevates the risk for bipolar disorder among veterans.

Dual Diagnosis and Comorbidity:

Veterans with bipolar disorder often experience comorbid mental health conditions, adding complexity to their overall well, being. Co, occurring conditions such as PTSD, substance use disorders, and anxiety disorders can interact with bipolar disorder symptoms, exacerbating mood episodes and complicating treatment outcomes. Mental health professionals working with veterans must adopt an integrated and holistic approach that addresses both bipolar disorder and any co, occurring conditions.

Trauma, Informed Care:

Given the prevalence of trauma among veterans, mental health professionals should adopt a trauma, informed care approach when treating individuals with bipolar disorder. This approach emphasizes safety, trustworthiness, choice, collaboration, and empowerment. Recognizing the impact of trauma on bipolar disorder symptoms and tailoring interventions to address past trauma can improve treatment outcomes and enhance overall well, being.

Suicide Risk and Prevention:

Veterans with bipolar disorder face an increased risk of suicide. The intersection of bipolar disorder, PTSD, and other mental health challenges creates a complex set of risk factors. Mental health professionals should conduct comprehensive suicide risk assessments and develop safety plans that address the specific needs and challenges faced by veterans. Close collaboration with support networks, such as veteran organizations and crisis helplines, is crucial in providing timely and effective interventions.

Medication Management and Side Effects:

Medication management plays a critical role in the treatment of bipolar disorder among veterans. However, it is essential to consider potential interactions with other medications and treatments commonly used in veterans' healthcare, such as those for PTSD or pain management. Mental health professionals should work closely with healthcare providers to ensure appropriate medication choices, monitor for potential side effects, and adjust treatment plans as necessary.

Access to Care and Veterans Affairs (VA) Services:

Access to mental health care is crucial for veterans with bipolar disorder. The Department of Veterans Affairs (VA) offers specialized mental health services tailored to the unique needs of veterans. Mental health professionals should be knowledgeable about VA services and eligibility criteria, ensuring that veterans receive the necessary support and treatments through VA programs. Collaborating with VA healthcare providers and coordinating care between VA and non, VA providers can optimize treatment outcomes.

Veteran Support Networks and Peer Support:

Engaging with veteran support networks and peer support programs can significantly benefit individuals with bipolar disorder. Veteran, specific support groups and organizations provide a sense of camaraderie, understanding, and validation. Peer support programs, facilitated by trained veterans who have lived experience with mental health challenges, offer a unique form of support and can enhance treatment adherence and recovery.

The impact of military service on mental health

The Silent Wounds: The Impact of Military Service on Mental Health

Military service is a noble and challenging profession that can have lasting effects on the mental health of those who serve. The unique experiences and stressors faced by service members can contribute to the development of mental health conditions, including bipolar disorder. This essay explores the impact of military service on mental health, shedding light on the risk factors, challenges, and considerations in relation to bipolar disorder.

Traumatic Experiences and Post, Traumatic Stress Disorder (PTSD):

Military personnel often face traumatic experiences during their service, such as combat exposure, witnessing violence, or experiencing life, threatening situations. These traumatic events can lead to the development of PTSD, a mental health condition characterized by intrusive thoughts, flashbacks, and hypervigilance. The co, occurrence of bipolar disorder and PTSD is not uncommon, and the combination can pose unique challenges for diagnosis and treatment.

Deployment and Separation:

Frequent deployments and prolonged periods of separation from loved ones can have a significant impact on mental health. The stress and emotional toll of being away from family and support networks can contribute to the development or exacerbation of mental health conditions, including bipolar disorder. The readjustment process upon returning from deployment can also be challenging and may lead to increased vulnerability to mood episodes.

High, Stress Environments and Psychological Demands:

Military environments are characterized by high levels of stress, strict discipline, and demanding responsibilities. These factors can place significant psychological burdens on service members, contributing to the development of mental health conditions. The unique demands of military service, such as operational tempo, long work hours, and exposure to life, threatening situations, can increase the risk of bipolar disorder among military personnel.

Stigma and Barriers to Seeking Help:

Stigma surrounding mental health issues remains a significant barrier to seeking help within the military culture. The perception of weakness, fear of negative career repercussions, and concerns about confidentiality may prevent service members from accessing necessary mental health support. Addressing stigma and promoting a culture of open dialogue and support are essential in creating an environment where service members feel comfortable seeking help for bipolar disorder and other mental health concerns.

Transitions and Reintegration:

The transition from military to civilian life can be a significant adjustment for service members. The loss of structure, identity, and social support networks can contribute to feelings of isolation, anxiety, and depression. These challenges can interact with bipolar disorder symptoms and increase the risk of mood episodes. Support during the transition process, including access to mental health services, vocational support, and peer networks, is crucial for a successful reintegration.

Co, occurring Substance Use Disorders:

Service members may be at increased risk of developing substance use disorders as a way to cope with the stressors and traumas associated with military service. Co, occurring substance use disorders and bipolar disorder can complicate diagnosis, treatment, and recovery. Mental health professionals working with military personnel should be aware of the potential interaction between bipolar disorder and substance use and address both conditions concurrently.

Suicide Risk and Prevention:

The risk of suicide is a significant concern among military personnel, particularly those with bipolar disorder. Multiple factors, including combat exposure, deployment, related stress, and untreated mental health conditions, contribute to increased suicide risk. Mental health professionals should be vigilant in assessing suicide risk, providing appropriate interventions, and promoting suicide prevention strategies within the military community.

Supportive Services and Resources:

Recognizing the impact of military service on mental health, the military provides a range of supportive services and resources. These include mental health clinics, counseling programs, peer support networks, and resilience training. Mental health professionals should collaborate with military healthcare providers, utilize available resources, and ensure service members are aware of the support services available to them.

Unique challenges faced by veterans with bipolar disorder

Hidden Battles: Unique Challenges Faced by Veterans with Bipolar Disorder

Bipolar disorder is a complex mental health condition that poses unique challenges for individuals, particularly for veterans who have served in the military. The intersection of bipolar disorder and the veteran experience creates a distinct set of challenges that impact the well, being and quality of life of those affected. This essay explores the unique challenges faced by veterans with bipolar disorder, shedding light on the impact of military service, access to care, stigma, and the importance of tailored support.

Military Service, Related Trauma:

Military service often exposes veterans to traumatic events that can contribute to the development of bipolar disorder. The experience of combat, witnessing violence, and exposure to life, threatening situations can significantly impact mental health. The interaction between bipolar disorder and trauma can intensify symptoms and complicate treatment, necessitating specialized care that addresses both the underlying condition and the military, related trauma.

Dual Diagnosis and Co, occurring Disorders:

Veterans with bipolar disorder frequently experience co, occurring mental health conditions, including post, traumatic stress disorder (PTSD), substance use disorders, and anxiety disorders. These comorbid conditions can exacerbate bipolar symptoms and create additional challenges for diagnosis and treatment. Mental health professionals must employ an integrated and comprehensive approach to address the complex needs of veterans with bipolar disorder and co, occurring disorders.

Treatment Accessibility and Availability:

Accessing appropriate mental health care can be a significant challenge for veterans with bipolar disorder. Limited resources, long wait times, and geographic barriers can impede timely access to care. Additionally, the stigma surrounding mental health issues within the military culture may deter veterans from seeking help. It is crucial to improve mental health care accessibility and availability, ensuring that veterans can access the specialized services they require.

Transition and Adjustment:

The transition from military to civilian life can be particularly challenging for veterans with bipolar disorder. Loss of structure, identity, and social support networks can exacerbate symptoms and contribute to feelings of isolation and anxiety. Adjusting to the civilian workforce, relationships, and daily routines requires ongoing support and understanding. Mental health professionals should address the unique challenges faced during the transition process, providing guidance and resources for a successful adjustment.

Employment and Vocational Challenges:

Bipolar disorder can impact employment and career stability for veterans. The unpredictable nature of the condition, including mood swings and episodes, may affect job performance and lead to challenges in maintaining employment. Veterans with bipolar disorder may require accommodations, vocational rehabilitation, and career counseling to achieve meaningful employment and financial stability.

Dual Identity and Stigma:

Veterans with bipolar disorder often grapple with the dual identity of being a veteran and living with a mental health condition. Stigma surrounding mental health issues can compound the challenges faced by veterans, creating barriers to seeking help and accessing support. Mental health professionals should address this unique dual identity, providing a safe and non, judgmental space for veterans to share their experiences and concerns.

Social Support and Peer Networks:

Building strong social support networks is crucial for veterans with bipolar disorder. Peer support programs, such as those offered by veteran organizations, provide a sense of camaraderie, understanding, and validation. Connecting veterans with bipolar disorder to peer networks and support groups fosters a sense of belonging and facilitates shared experiences and coping strategies.

Trauma, Informed Care:

Trauma, informed care is vital for veterans with bipolar disorder, given the prevalence of military, related trauma. Mental health professionals should adopt an approach that acknowledges the impact of trauma, prioritizes safety and trust, and empowers veterans in their treatment journey. Providing trauma, informed care promotes healing, resilience, and improved mental health outcomes.

Resources and support for veterans and their families

Healing the Wounds: Resources and Support for Veterans and Their Families

Veterans and their families often face unique challenges related to mental health, particularly when navigating conditions like bipolar disorder. Access to comprehensive resources and support services is crucial for promoting the well, being and recovery of both veterans and their loved ones. This essay explores the available resources and support systems tailored to meet the needs of veterans and their families, with a specific focus on bipolar disorder and its impact on mental health.

Department of Veterans Affairs (VA) Services:

The Department of Veterans Affairs offers a wide range of mental health services specifically designed for veterans. These services may include counseling, psychiatric care, medication management, and residential treatment programs. The VA's specialized care for mental health conditions, including bipolar disorder, ensures that veterans receive tailored support from professionals with expertise in military, related mental health issues.

Vet Centers:

Vet Centers are community, based counseling centers that provide free and confidential counseling services to combat veterans and their families. These centers offer individual, group, and family counseling, as well as referrals to additional resources. Vet Centers provide a safe and supportive environment for veterans and their families to address the challenges associated with bipolar disorder and other mental health conditions.

National Alliance on Mental Illness (NAMI):

NAMI is a leading organization that provides education, support, and advocacy for individuals and families affected by mental health conditions. NAMI offers various programs and resources specifically tailored to veterans and their families, including support groups, educational workshops, and helpline services. NAMI's peer, led support groups, in particular, provide a space for veterans and their families to connect with others who understand their unique experiences.

Military OneSource:

Military OneSource is a comprehensive resource that offers a range of services to support military families. Their services include non, medical counseling, financial counseling, legal assistance, and access to confidential support 24/ Military OneSource can provide valuable guidance and assistance to veterans and their families in navigating the challenges associated with bipolar disorder and accessing appropriate care.

TRICARE Mental Health Coverage:

TRICARE is the health care program for uniformed service members, retirees, and their families. TRICARE offers mental health coverage, including outpatient therapy, inpatient treatment, and medication management for bipolar disorder and other mental health conditions. Veterans and their families can access mental health services through TRICARE, ensuring comprehensive and affordable care.

Family Support Programs:

Recognizing the impact of mental health conditions on family dynamics, several programs specifically target support for the families of veterans. The Family, to, Family program offered by NAMI provides education, resources, and support for families caring for loved ones with mental health conditions. Additionally, caregiver support programs, such as those offered by the VA, aim to alleviate the challenges faced by family members caring for veterans with bipolar disorder.

Online Support Networks:

Virtual support networks provide accessible and convenient resources for veterans and their families. Websites and online communities dedicated to supporting veterans and promoting mental health offer valuable information, discussion forums, and resources. These platforms connect individuals with shared experiences, fostering a sense of community and reducing feelings of isolation.

Peer Support and Veteran Organizations:

Peer support programs and veteran organizations play a critical role in connecting veterans and their families with support networks. Organizations such as the Wounded Warrior Project, Iraq and Afghanistan Veterans of America (IAVA), and Veterans of Foreign Wars (VFW) offer resources, advocacy, and opportunities for peer, to, peer support. Connecting with these organizations allows veterans and their families to engage with others who have similar experiences and challenges.

Chapter Thirty-One

Personal Stories and Memoirs

Illuminating Journeys: Personal Stories and Memoirs of Bipolar Disorder

Personal stories and memoirs have the power to shed light on the lived experiences of individuals with bipolar disorder. These narratives offer a unique window into the challenges, triumphs, and resilience of those affected by the condition. By sharing their personal journeys, individuals with bipolar disorder can provide insight, inspiration, and a sense of community for others facing similar struggles. This essay explores the significance of personal stories and memoirs in relation to bipolar disorder, highlighting their ability to educate, reduce stigma, and foster empathy.

Raising Awareness and Education:

Personal stories and memoirs serve as powerful educational tools for understanding bipolar disorder. By sharing their experiences, individuals can provide firsthand accounts of the symptoms, challenges, and treatment of the condition. These narratives help demystify bipolar disorder and provide valuable insights into the day, to, day realities faced by those living with the condition. Personal stories can also dispel misconceptions and promote accurate understanding among the general public.

Breaking Down Stigma:

Stigma surrounding mental health conditions, including bipolar disorder, often leads to shame, discrimination, and isolation. Personal stories and memoirs act as catalysts for breaking down these barriers. They humanize the condition by sharing personal triumphs, setbacks, and vulnerabilities, helping others recognize the shared humanity in individuals with bipolar disorder. By challenging stereotypes and fostering empathy, personal stories contribute to reducing stigma and fostering a more inclusive society.

Empowering Individuals:

Personal stories and memoirs have the power to empower individuals with bipolar disorder. By sharing their journeys of self, discovery, treatment, and resilience, individuals inspire others to seek help, persevere, and embrace their own personal growth. These stories remind individuals that they are not alone and that recovery and meaningful lives are possible despite the challenges posed by bipolar disorder. By highlighting personal strengths and strategies for coping, personal narratives instill hope and motivation in others.

Providing Validation and Connection:

Reading personal stories and memoirs can provide a profound sense of validation and connection for individuals with bipolar disorder. When individuals see their own experiences reflected in the stories of others, they realize they are not alone in their struggles. Personal narratives offer a sense of belonging and understanding, fostering a supportive community for individuals to share their own stories and find solace in the shared journey of bipolar disorder.

Offering Insights for Loved Ones:

Personal stories and memoirs also provide valuable insights for the loved ones of individuals with bipolar disorder. These narratives offer a glimpse into the emotional rollercoaster, challenges with treatment adherence, and impact on relationships that loved ones may not fully comprehend. By gaining a deeper understanding of the experiences of individuals with bipolar disorder, family members and friends can provide better support and navigate their own emotional journey.

Diverse Perspectives:

Personal stories and memoirs highlight the diversity of experiences within the bipolar community. Each individual's journey is unique, influenced by factors such as age, gender, cultural background, and socioeconomic status. Personal narratives offer a range of perspectives, enabling readers to recognize the nuances of living with bipolar disorder and appreciate the intersectionality of identities and experiences.

Inspiring Advocacy and Change:

Personal stories and memoirs often serve as catalysts for advocacy and social change. By sharing their experiences, individuals with bipolar disorder raise awareness, promote policy reform, and advocate for improved mental health services. These narratives humanize the issues faced by individuals with bipolar disorder, compelling policymakers, healthcare providers, and the general public to prioritize mental health care and support systems.

First

,

hand accounts of living with bipolar disorder

Illuminating the Human Experience: First, Hand Accounts of Living with Bipolar Disorder

First, hand accounts of individuals living with bipolar disorder offer invaluable insights into the complex and multifaceted nature of the condition. These personal narratives go beyond clinical descriptions, providing a human perspective on the daily challenges, triumphs, and resilience of those navigating bipolar disorder. By sharing their lived experiences, individuals with bipolar disorder not only increase awareness but also foster empathy, reduce stigma, and provide hope to others facing similar journeys. This essay explores the significance of first, hand accounts in relation to bipolar disorder, highlighting their impact on understanding, support, and personal growth.

Unique Perspectives:

First, hand accounts capture the diversity of experiences within the bipolar community. Each individual's journey with bipolar disorder is shaped by personal factors such as age, gender, cultural background, and socioeconomic status. These narratives offer a range of perspectives, reflecting the complexity and individuality of living with bipolar disorder. By sharing their stories, individuals provide readers with a deeper understanding of the condition's nuanced impact on their lives.

Embracing Vulnerability:

Sharing personal experiences of living with bipolar disorder requires immense vulnerability. These narratives delve into the emotional highs and lows, the challenges of managing relationships, and the impact of treatment. By openly discussing their vulnerabilities, individuals with bipolar disorder break down barriers and inspire others to embrace their own journey with authenticity and self, acceptance.

Breaking Down Stigma:

Stigma surrounding mental health conditions can be isolating and deter individuals from seeking help. First, hand accounts challenge stigma by humanizing bipolar disorder and dispelling misconceptions. By sharing their personal stories, individuals confront societal stereotypes and promote understanding, compassion, and acceptance. These narratives encourage open conversations about mental health, fostering an environment where individuals feel safe and supported.

Empathy and Connection:

First, hand accounts of living with bipolar disorder foster empathy and connection. Readers who have not experienced the condition firsthand gain insight into the emotional rollercoaster, the challenges of treatment adherence, and the impact on relationships. By sharing their vulnerabilities and triumphs, individuals with bipolar disorder create a sense of community, allowing others to connect, relate, and find solace in the shared experiences of living with the condition.

Offering Practical Insights:

Personal narratives provide practical insights for individuals with bipolar disorder and their loved ones. They offer coping strategies, self, care tips, and reflections on navigating treatment and recovery. These practical insights, rooted in personal experiences, provide readers with a deeper understanding of what works and what doesn't in managing bipolar disorder. Such insights empower individuals to make informed decisions about their own treatment and well, being.

Navigating Relationships:

First, hand accounts shed light on the impact of bipolar disorder on relationships with family, friends, and romantic partners. Individuals share their experiences of navigating the challenges, including communication difficulties, mood fluctuations, and the need for understanding and support. These narratives offer guidance for loved ones, helping them develop empathy, patience, and strategies for maintaining healthy and supportive relationships.

Inspiration and Hope:

Personal narratives inspire and instill hope in individuals facing bipolar disorder. By sharing their stories of resilience, personal growth, and successful management of the condition, individuals provide encouragement to others. These narratives remind readers that recovery is possible and that a fulfilling and meaningful life can be achieved despite the challenges of bipolar disorder. They offer hope during difficult times and inspire individuals to seek help, explore treatment options, and embrace a journey of personal growth.

Advocacy and Awareness:

First, hand accounts of living with bipolar disorder often spur advocacy efforts and contribute to increased awareness. Individuals who share their stories become advocates for mental health, calling for improved resources, increased access to treatment, and reduced stigma.

Overcoming adversity and finding hope

Illuminating the Path: Overcoming Adversity and Finding Hope in Bipolar Disorder

Bipolar disorder is a complex mental health condition that presents numerous challenges, but it is also a journey marked by resilience, personal growth, and the discovery of hope. Individuals living with bipolar disorder often encounter significant adversity, including emotional ups and downs, treatment setbacks, and societal stigma. However, many individuals have managed to overcome these obstacles and find hope amidst their struggles. This essay explores the stories of resilience and hope in the context of bipolar disorder, highlighting the transformative power of self, acceptance, support systems, and a positive outlook.

Embracing Self, Acceptance:

Overcoming adversity in bipolar disorder begins with self, acceptance. Individuals who have found hope have often reached a point of acknowledging and accepting their diagnosis. By embracing their condition as a part of their identity, they are empowered to take control of their mental health and make informed decisions about treatment and self, care. Self, acceptance allows individuals to focus on their strengths, build resilience, and navigate the challenges of bipolar disorder with a sense of purpose and self, assuredness.

Building a Support System:

Finding hope often involves seeking and nurturing a support system. Whether it be family, friends, support groups, or mental health professionals, individuals with bipolar disorder who have overcome adversity have recognized the importance of a strong support network. These networks offer understanding, encouragement, and practical assistance during challenging times. Support systems provide validation, create a sense of belonging, and offer a safe space to share experiences and emotions.

Treatment and Therapy:

Successful navigation of bipolar disorder involves finding effective treatment and therapy options. Individuals who have found hope in their journey have actively engaged in treatment modalities such as medication, therapy, and lifestyle adjustments. They have collaborated with mental health professionals to develop personalized strategies for managing symptoms and promoting stability. By actively participating in treatment, individuals gain a sense of agency and control over their mental health, leading to improved overall well, being.

Resilience and Coping Strategies:

Resilience plays a crucial role in overcoming adversity in bipolar disorder. Individuals who have found hope have developed effective coping strategies to manage the challenges that arise. These strategies may include mindfulness practices, exercise, creative outlets, journaling, or engaging in hobbies. By nurturing their resilience and implementing healthy coping mechanisms, individuals with bipolar disorder can navigate mood swings, stress, and setbacks with greater ease and resilience.

Seeking Meaning and Purpose:

Finding hope often involves seeking meaning and purpose in life. Individuals with bipolar disorder who have overcome adversity have discovered ways to cultivate a sense of meaning, whether through creative pursuits, volunteer work, advocacy, or engaging in meaningful relationships. Finding purpose provides individuals with a sense of fulfillment and motivation, helping them weather the storms of bipolar disorder and remain focused on their personal growth and aspirations.

Positive Mindset and Gratitude:

Maintaining a positive mindset and practicing gratitude can significantly impact one's journey with bipolar disorder. Individuals who have found hope have developed a positive outlook, focusing on the possibilities and strengths rather than the limitations imposed by their condition. Cultivating gratitude for small victories and embracing a positive mindset allows individuals to reframe challenges as opportunities for growth and learning, fostering resilience and hope.

Redefining Success:

Overcoming adversity in bipolar disorder often involves redefining what success means. Individuals who have found hope have shifted their focus from external achievements to personal well, being and self, fulfillment. They recognize that success encompasses emotional stability, healthy relationships, personal growth, and self, care, rather than conforming to societal expectations. By redefining success, individuals with bipolar disorder can celebrate their progress and find fulfillment in their unique journey.

Lessons learned and insights gained from personal experiences

Wisdom Through Experience: Lessons Learned and Insights Gained from Personal Experiences with Bipolar Disorder

Personal experiences with bipolar disorder offer invaluable lessons and insights into the complexities of living with this mental health condition. Individuals who have navigated the highs and lows of bipolar disorder have acquired a wealth of wisdom that can enlighten and guide others on their own journeys. This essay explores the lessons learned and insights gained from personal experiences, highlighting the importance of self, awareness, resilience, self, care, and the pursuit of holistic well, being.

The Power of Self, Awareness:

Personal experiences with bipolar disorder underscore the significance of self, awareness. Individuals who have journeyed through the condition have developed a deep understanding of their triggers, symptoms, and warning signs. By recognizing their own patterns, they are better equipped to anticipate and manage mood fluctuations. Self, awareness enables individuals to make informed decisions about their treatment, lifestyle choices, and overall well, being.

Embracing the Spectrum of Emotions:

Living with bipolar disorder exposes individuals to a wide spectrum of emotions, ranging from the depths of despair to the heights of euphoria. Personal experiences emphasize the importance of acknowledging and accepting these emotions without judgment. Rather than viewing emotions as inherently negative or positive, individuals learn to navigate and embrace the richness and complexity of their emotional landscape.

Resilience and Adaptability:

Personal experiences with bipolar disorder highlight the resilience and adaptability of individuals in the face of adversity. Individuals learn to bounce back from setbacks, manage daily challenges, and adapt their coping strategies as needed. Through resilience, individuals with bipolar disorder demonstrate their capacity to overcome obstacles and find strength in times of difficulty.

The Importance of Self, Care:

Personal experiences underscore the critical role of self, care in managing bipolar disorder. Individuals learn that self, care is not a luxury but a necessity for maintaining stability and well, being. Strategies such as establishing consistent sleep patterns, practicing mindfulness, engaging in regular exercise, maintaining a balanced diet, and cultivating meaningful relationships all contribute to overall wellness and help mitigate the impact of bipolar disorder.

Holistic Approaches to Well, Being:

Living with bipolar disorder encourages individuals to adopt a holistic approach to well, being that encompasses physical, emotional, and spiritual aspects of life. Personal experiences often reveal the value of engaging in activities that promote balance, such as creative expression, connecting with nature, engaging in hobbies, and finding meaning through spiritual practices. Taking care of one's mental health extends beyond medical interventions to include activities that nourish the soul and foster a sense of purpose.

Building a Supportive Network:

Personal experiences highlight the importance of building a supportive network of family, friends, and mental health professionals. Individuals learn to seek out those who understand and validate their experiences, providing invaluable emotional support. Supportive relationships offer a safe space for open communication, empathy, and understanding, reducing the sense of isolation often associated with bipolar disorder.

Navigating Medication and Treatment Options:

Personal experiences shed light on the complexities of medication and treatment management for bipolar disorder. Individuals learn that finding the right combination of medications and therapies can be a journey of trial and error. Through personal experiences, individuals gain insight into the importance of open communication with healthcare providers, advocating for their needs, and actively participating in their treatment plan.

The Importance of Boundaries and Self, Advocacy:

Living with bipolar disorder often necessitates the establishment of boundaries and assertive self, advocacy. Personal experiences highlight the importance of setting limits on activities, relationships, and responsibilities to protect one's well, being. Individuals learn to assert their needs, communicate boundaries effectively, and prioritize self, care without guilt or shame.

* 9 7 8 1 7 7 6 8 4 7 0 3 7 *
SD - #0018 - 140926 - C0 - 229/152/19 - PB - 9781776847037 - Matt Lamination